About the Author

Jon S. Abramson received his undergraduate degree at Boston University and medical degree from Wake Forest School of Medicine (WFSM). He did a pediatric residency at Wake Forest Baptist Medical Center and pediatric infectious diseases fellowship at the University of Minnesota. He joined the faculty at WFSM in 1981 and served as Chair of the Department of Pediatrics at WFSM and Physician-in-Chief of Brenner Children's Hospital from June 1996 – June 2014. In 2017, his status changed to Professor Emeritus. During the past decade he has worked with the World Health Organization (WHO), Global Alliance for Vaccines and Immunization (Gavi) and other global partner organizations on issues related to vaccines and immunization programs.

Published by

World Scientific Publishing Co. Pte. Ltd.

5 Toh Tuck Link, Singapore 596224

USA office: 27 Warren Street, Suite 401-402, Hackensack, NJ 07601

UK office: 57 Shelton Street, Covent Garden, London WC2H 9HE

British Library Cataloguing-in-Publication Data
A catalogue record for this book is available from the British Library.

OVERWHELMED
A Tale of Cascading Viral Outbreaks

ISBN 978-981-124-034-8 (hardcover)
ISBN 978-981-123-858-1 (paperback)
ISBN 978-981-123-859-8 (ebook for institutions)
ISBN 978-981-123-860-4 (ebook for individuals)

For any available supplementary material, please visit
https://www.worldscientific.com/worldscibooks/10.1142/12322#t=suppl

Foreword

The inspiration for this novel comes from actual infectious disease outbreaks that occurred during this past decade. While the medical discussions in the book are based on real events, the scenes and characters are fictional.

Dedication

To all those providing care to people affected by infectious disease outbreaks.

Prologue

Since the beginning of the 21st century, the world has been experiencing one infectious disease outbreak after another, with little time to breathe between events. Now, in the first quarter of 2020, a new strain of coronavirus (SARS-CoV-2), first detected in China, is causing a worldwide pandemic. Health care systems in many countries are in danger of being overrun and care for many of those who are sick occurs in provisional settings. Intensive care units have exceeded their normal capacity and healthcare workers are doing their best to provide care in a chaotic environment. This situation is exacerbated by an inadequate supply of protective gowns, masks and other equipment: as well as a shortage of healthcare workers who have been infected by the virus. The World Health Organization (WHO) is overseeing intense efforts to develop and test drugs and vaccines that can treat or prevent COVID-19 disease. However, even when identified, there will be insufficient quantities of these items available for the global population for months to years. Vital infrastructure services remain functional in many countries, but the negative economic impact of the pandemic is having a severe impact on many people.

The warning signs that a pandemic was coming had been there for years. The WHO leadership received harsh criticism for their handling of the Ebola crisis in 2014, and responded by creating a visionary blueprint plan to guide their responses to new infectious disease outbreaks. The WHO Director-General intensely lobbied countries for increased funding to support the plan, noting the four-fold increase in infectious disease outbreaks during the past decade and knowing that four influenza pandemics occurred during the previous century. Despite these pleas, many of the political leaders in wealthy countries were shifting from a global to a nationalistic focus and unwilling to donate the necessary funding to implement the entire plan. The outbreaks continue unabated and the COVID-19 pandemic is now upon us. It did not have to be this way.

Abbreviations

BSL — Biosafety laboratory
CDC — Centers for Disease Control and Prevention
COVID-19 — the name of the current pandemic
DRC — Democratic Republic of the Congo
Gavi — Global Alliance for Vaccines and Immunization
H — Hemagglutinin protein on the outer membrane of influenza viruses
MERS — Middle East Respiratory Syndrome
MSF — Médecins Sans Frontières (also known as Doctors without Borders)
N — Neuraminidase protein on the outer membrane of influenza viruses
SAGE — Strategic Advisory Group of Experts on Immunization
SARS-CoV-2 — Severe Acute Respiratory Syndrome Coronavirus-2
UN — United Nations
US — United States
WHO — World Health Organization

Contents

Chapter 1

Democratic Republic of the Congo
April 2016

The medical center is located in a rural area north of the Democratic Republic of the Congo (DRC) capital, Kinshasa that lies along the portion of the Congo River separating the DRC and Republic of the Congo, and is close to Angola's northern border. Yellow fever is running rampant through the DRC. As Dr. David Ferguson enters the Kuzi medical center, he cannot help but think about how this yellow fever outbreak is worse than any other he has seen in the past decades working in various countries for the World Health Organization (WHO).

This yellow fever outbreak is threatening to overwhelm all their efforts to control the spread of the disease, including mosquito control and vaccinating the population. During the past few weeks, the number of people seeking care has increased from around 30 to over 70 per day. Some patients are in the first phase of their illness with flu-like symptoms and are being cared for in the outpatient clinic, but others have progressed to a toxic second phase that requires admission to the makeshift hospital consisting of four temporary tents connected to a storage building that serves as the central hub.

During the first month of the outbreak, each of the four hospital tents contained 5–10 patients, cared for by a nurse and a healthcare assistant. Now there are often 20 patients in each wing and most patients have a family member with them at the bedside. To make matters worse, the outside temperature for this past week has exceeded 30°C (86°F) every day and the humidity has been high. The weather, along with the crowded conditions, results in a strong musty smell inside the hospital that never seems to go away. The number of healthcare staff is inadequate for the increasing number of patients and everyone is exhausted.

David is in the hospital helping Aceline Durand who works for Médecins Sans Frontières (MSF), a non-profit international humanitarian organization providing routine and emergency medical healthcare care in developing countries. They are caring for Egbeble, a 12-year-old boy, admitted to the hospital an hour ago with delirium and bleeding from his nose and mouth. His eyes and skin are yellow, indicating the virus is affecting his liver and causing jaundice. Egbeble has pulled out his intravenous line and Aceline is struggling to put in another line so that they can continue to provide the fluids he needs. David looks over to Egbeble's parents who are by his bedside and asks in French, "How long has Egbeble been sick?"

The parents do not understand what David is saying and Aceline, who speaks several of the local dialects, repeats the question in Kikongo, a second national language in the DRC along with French. The father, Kasamba, responds, "Egbeble and I were in the jungle near our village hunting for food about a week ago. Three days after returning home, he started to become ill."

Aceline asks, "What was he complaining about?"

"Egbeble ached all over, felt hot, was shaking and did not want to eat. A few days later, his fever went away and he began to feel better. However, his fever came back yesterday and he started bleeding from his mouth this morning. Do you know what is wrong with Egbeble? Does he have malaria?"

"He likely has yellow fever. We sent a small amount of his blood to the laboratory in Kinshasa to test for this and a few other diseases."

Tangu, Egbeble's mother, replies, "Several people in a village near us developed yellow fever and one died. Will Egbeble be okay?"

Aceline finally gets a new intravenous line established and turns towards Tangu. "Most people with yellow fever get chills and aches as Egbeble had, but then recover within a week. However, Egbeble's fever has reoccurred and it seems he has gone on to the second stage, which is more dangerous."

Tears form in Kasamba's eyes as he gasps, "Will he die?" Aceline knows there is no specific treatment for yellow fever and while the mortality rate is around 10% overall, approximately 50% of the patients who progress onto the more toxic second stage, die. She turns to David and quickly tells him the gist of the conversation.

David responds, "Just tell them that most of those who are admitted to the hospital with yellow fever recover and go home."

Aceline glares at David. "I will NOT tell them that. I am not going to overpromise."

She then looks at the parents and quietly speaks, "We will do everything we can to help Egbeble. How are your other children doing?"

Tangu answers, "When we left the village this morning they seemed to be doing fine."

Aceline smiles. "That's good to hear. Has anyone come to your village to offer the yellow fever vaccine?"

"We heard people in another village were getting the yellow fever shot, but no one has come to our village."

"Would one of you be willing to travel with me tomorrow so that we can talk to people in your village about getting the vaccine?" Aceline asks.

Tangu volunteers. "I will go with you. I want to check on my other children and make sure they are okay."

"Where is your village located and how difficult will it be to get there?"

"We live in the Equator region. It took us over six hours to bring Egbeble here from our village. We had to walk to get to the river and then took a boat down to the medical center," says Kasamba.

Aceline inquires, "Once we get off the boat, can we take a vehicle to get to the village?"

Kasamba answers, "The jungle area you must go through can only be reached by motorcycle or walking."

Aceline turns to David. "Can you get someone to make arrangements for the boat ride and motorcycle drivers to help us get to the village with the vaccine supplies?" David nods.

Aceline looks back at Tangu. "Tomorrow I will pick you up here at sunrise."

David knows they have done all they can for Egbeble for now. He thinks Aceline is mad at him and decides they should talk. David smiles at her. "Let's get some lunch and you can critique my bedside manner."

"I need a shower first. I will meet you in the mess tent in 30 minutes."

David goes back to his office and his thoughts drift to when Aceline and he first met. He has worked for the WHO for 12 years on various public health emergencies, including outbreaks of cholera in Africa, avian influenza in Asia and the Middle East, and yellow fever in central Africa. Most recently, he was in Liberia during the 2014 Western Africa Ebola virus outbreak, which is where he first met Aceline. He had been overseeing the WHO response and she was doing the same for the MSF.

They spent a lot of time together while in Liberia (and now in the DRC), both during and after work. Initially, he thought she was in her mid-20s, but along the way, learned she was closer to his age. Aceline was born in France in 1980 to missionary parents, and during her childhood lived in various African countries. She returned to France just after her 18th birthday to obtain a nursing degree and then started working as an emergency department nurse at a large hospital in Marseille. She got married soon after taking this job, but this eventually ended in divorce a decade later. Thereafter, she decided to pursue a career doing humanitarian medical work in Africa and accepted a position with MSF. For the past decade, she has provided care to children and adults in different African countries during various infectious disease outbreaks.

David admires Aceline's intelligence and her excellent clinical, organizational, and leadership skills. These qualities were once again evident in helping her oversee the MSF and Congolese staff working with them on the current yellow fever outbreak in the DRC.

He also has developed romantic feelings for Aceline during their time together and hopes the relationship can move beyond their current friendship. He wonders if the feeling is reciprocal since at times, like today, she seems to find some of his actions infuriating.

He walks over to the mess tent and she is there waiting for him. While eating lunch, he apologizes for asking her to tell Egbeble's parents something that was not correct. "Your response to Egbeble's parents' question about his chance of dying was much better than my suggestion."

"David, you are an excellent physician and do a great job overseeing the medical center. However, sometimes you need to be more perceptive about what you say to those around you."

"I thought the parents wouldn't be able to handle the fact that Egbeble had a 50% chance of dying.

Aceline reaches her hand across the table and puts it on his forearm. "I did not give them a percentage. What I told them was that we would do everything we could for him. This is a much better way to help comfort them without giving them false hope."

"Your ability to communicate is one of the many things I admire about you."

Before they can finish their conversation, Atazia, a nurse working in the hospital, comes to their table and informs Aceline that Bonte, the Congolese healthcare aid she works with, was just stuck with a needle used to draw blood from a patient. David and Aceline immediately get up from the table and go with Atazia to see Bonte.

Bonte is sitting outside the hospital tent and Aceline sees the fear expressed on his face. "Bonte, please tell us what happened."

Bonte stutters while speaking rapidly, "Atazia and I were trying to do a blood test on a patient who was hallucinating. I was holding the patient's arm in place and just as Atazia was getting blood back from the vein, the patient became very combative and pushed the needle into my hand."

Aceline asks, "What do we know about this patient?"

Bonte replies, "His test came back positive for yellow fever yesterday. Am I going to get yellow fever?"

David chimes in, "You and all the other healthcare workers here received the vaccine that will protect you from getting yellow fever. However, we still have to check for some other diseases."

Bonte is even more concerned now. "Will I get HIV?"

David responds, "We will test the patient's blood for HIV. If the test is negative, we will not need to do anything else. We can do the HIV test in our on-site laboratory and will know the answer later today."

Aceline adds, "Bonte, we know you are worried. Please take the rest of the afternoon off and I will get one of the other workers to cover your patients."

Bonte fearfully stares at both of them. "I will be back later today to find out about the HIV test."

Aceline and David head back to finish lunch. She is concerned about the heavy workload the medical staff is taking on. "The staff is overburdened with too many patients. They are all doing double shifts and some have not had a day off in over two weeks. The number of accidents like Bonte's will get worse unless we can get more staff here."

David, knowing this is true, replies, "I will ask all the staff that can make themselves available to come to a short meeting in the cafeteria. We can reinforce the need to follow all safety protocols and hear from them about how else we can support them."

Thirty minutes later, they meet with the staff. The meeting is very tense and goes on longer than expected. It is clear from the conversation that the number one concern of the healthcare staff is getting more help. Towards the end of the meeting, one of them stands up and says, "You promised us more help last week and nothing has happened. We don't want to turn away anyone who is sick, but more help must be found." David praises them for the care they are providing under very trying circumstances and once again promises to do everything he can to find them more staff by the end of the week.

David goes back to his office and for the third time this month, calls the WHO's DRC office in Kinshasa asking for more staff and supplies. He learns they hope they can get him what he needs early next week, but their current focus is on determining whether a patient admitted yesterday to a hospital in Kinshasa who never traveled outside the city has yellow fever.

David throws his cell phone onto his desk in defeat and then collapses into his chair. Kinshasa has a population of over ten million people and a large infestation of Aedes mosquitoes capable of transmitting the yellow fever virus from one person to another. The expansion of the yellow fever outbreak into this urban area could result in the infection of many of those living in the city and high numbers of deaths.

Aceline walks into David's office and sees that he looks despondent. "Please tell me they can get us more help and supplies."

David looks at her. "They hope they can get us both by next week, but there may be an even bigger problem." He tells her what he learned about a possible case of yellow fever in Kinshasa.

Aceline becomes agitated and says exasperatedly, "We don't have enough staff to vaccinate everyone in our rural area. A mass vaccination campaign that includes Kinshasa will require millions of additional doses of the vaccine and hundreds of additional healthcare workers. You tell me how we are going to find them?"

David understands her anger is not directed towards him. "We both need to get some sleep. We can talk tomorrow when you get back from Egbeble's village. Hopefully, I will know more about the possible case in Kinshasa by then."

***

Just before sunrise, Aceline meets up with Tangu who is sitting by Egbeble's bed. Aceline asks the nurse if there has been any change in his condition and she shake her head no. Aceline then asks Tangu if she is still willing to travel to her village and she nods "yes". They, along with a medical center staff member familiar with the area around Egbeble's village, walk a short distance to the Congo River where a boat is waiting.

The Congo River functions as the main route of transportation in the DRC where dense forests are common and paved roads are few. The breeze feels good as they travel along the river on what is already becoming another hot and humid day. Aceline has taken many boat trips on the Congo River, but always finds new things to observe. On this trip, she sees a variety of animals including leopards, lions, hyenas, and rhinoceroses. She also sees a bulbul, a type of songbird that is abundant in the DRC, but this one has orange coloring, which is unusual since most bulbuls are completely black. Even after living in the DRC for years, Aceline is in awe of the animals in this country.

Aceline spends some time talking with Egbeble's mom about her family and the village they live in. She learns Egbeble is the oldest of her children. He does well in school and loves to hunt with his dad, play soccer, and carve wood into animal figures. His brother and sister, as well as many of the other children in the village, look up to him.

Their village is about 7 km from the river. There are 22 families living there and Muteba, Egbeble's paternal grandfather, is the leader. Their main sources of food come from farming and fishing. Normally, they receive their medical care by walking to an outpatient center located 3 km from the village. Most of the families get vaccines as part of their routine health care.

For the rest of the boat trip, Aceline's thoughts drift to her interactions with David. Aceline is very attracted to David, particularly his curly brown hair, trimmed beard, hazel eyes, and muscular build. During the two years they have worked together, her feelings for him have grown stronger and she believes he has similar feelings. However, separating their work relationship from their growing friendship is complicated and she feels there is a lot that remains unspoken between them.

She believes David's family background contributes a lot to who he is. He spent his childhood in rural northern Australia where his parents were physicians who worked to improve the health of the indigenous Aboriginal population. He was very close to his parents and knew at a relatively early age that he wanted to become a physician and work with disadvantaged populations. After graduating from the University of Queensland School Of Medicine in Australia, he moved to England to attend the London School of Hygiene and Tropical Medicine where he obtained a Master's degree in Public Health and Policy. He is smart, hardworking and has the ability to make quick assessments and implement effective solutions. She admires his dedication to improving global health. His parents died in an automobile accident soon after he started working for the WHO. Aceline wonders how much this tragedy still affects him and whether it inhibits his ability to express his feelings to her.

Upon leaving the boat, three drivers with motorbikes are waiting to take them along with their supplies through the jungle and dirt roads to the village. The motorbike ride takes several hours due to large potholes and impassable areas that require them to get off their bikes and walk. As they enter the village, Aceline sees about two dozen huts in an area where the jungle used to be. Some of the children in the village are playing with a worn soccer ball on a dirt field with puddles and potholes. Egbeble's brother and sister see their mother and run to greet her and ask about Egbeble. She tells them he is still sick and how glad she is to see that they look well.

They go to the family's hut and the first thing Aceline notices is that there are no mosquito nets over the beds. "Has the village been given any mosquito bed nets to protect against malaria?"

Tangu responds, "Yes, but Muteba thinks it is more important to use the nets to catch fish."

Aceline knows that only about half of the bed nets given to African villages are used for their intended purpose. Most people living in areas with malaria are aware the nets help decrease the number of cases of malaria, but do not prevent all cases of malaria. Some village leaders, such as Muteba, believe using the nets for fishing and clothing serve a better purpose.

Aceline asks, "Can we go meet Muteba?"

Tangu nods and walks with Aceline to his hut. Tangu introduces Aceline to Muteba and then tells him that Egbeble was admitted to the hospital with yellow fever and that Aceline is helping care for him.

Muteba looks at Aceline and asks, "How is Egbeble doing?" She notes the sadness on his face. "We are doing everything we can to help him get over his illness."

Muteba thinks for a moment and then replies, "I have lived through several yellow fever outbreaks and watched some of our people die. During these outbreaks, some of our healers used local remedies to try to heal those who became ill, but I do not think they helped. Is there something you can do to help protect our village?"

Aceline looks directly at Muteba. "Actually, yes. I have brought a vaccine that can prevent people from getting yellow fever. The protection from the vaccine lasts for a very long time and those who get the vaccine will be protected against the current and future yellow fever outbreaks."

"I have heard about this vaccine from people in other villages — they say it is good. I will tell everyone that they should get it."

Aceline thanks him. "We will set up in the middle of the village and give the vaccine to everyone who comes."

Aceline and her co-worker finish vaccinating everyone in the village just before dusk, but now it is too late to return to their healthcare center. Tangu invites them to sleep in their hut and they gladly accept the offer.

***

Upon their return to the medical center the following day, Tangu rushes to see Egbeble while Aceline goes to find David. David's face lights up when he sees her. "I was worried when you did not come back last night."

She sits down in the chair on the other side of his desk. "I would have called, but my cell phone had no reception in the village. I appreciate your concern, but right now I want to apologize for yelling at you before I left."

David grins. "Keeping our sanity demands a vent session at times. In fact, your response is in line with one of my three rules for keeping your sanity when everything is spiraling out of control."

Aceline gazes at David and gets a little distracted by the way she feels when he smiles. "I can't wait to hear your rules."

"I'll share them with you, but then you need to consider the rules when I tell you something that I just found out."

"First, when all your hard work blows up in your face, it usually is not your fault."

"Next, when bad things happen, laughing, screaming or crying is an appropriate response. This helps you to deal with your feelings more rapidly and move onto what needs to be done next. Sometimes, I do more than one."

"Finally, when we help others, we also help ourselves."

She laughs. "I like the rules, but now you have me worried about what you just learned."

He sighs. "The patient in Kinshasa tested positive for yellow fever and now they think they may have another case in the city."

She stares at him in disbelief. "Yellow fever was confined mainly to jungle areas in the past. What has changed?"

David knows the answer to her question is complex. "During the last several decades, climate change has enabled the geographical spread of the Aedes mosquito into new areas, including large urban settings. At the same time, there is a greater migration of people traveling from rural areas into urban areas. In this area, the migrant population moves back and forth across the border between the DRC and Angola looking for work in Kinshasa. The native population in Kinshasa and other urban areas are at high risk for yellow fever since most of the population are susceptible to the virus and have not been vaccinated."

Aceline is furious. "The yellow fever vaccine has been available for many decades at a low cost. Given the number of previous yellow fever outbreaks in the DRC, it is infuriating the vaccine is not more widely used in this country. How many new outbreaks will have to occur before this is done?"

David admires her passion. "I share your outrage."

Aceline takes a minute to calm down and decides it is time to change the topic. "I'm going over to see Egbeble, do you know how he is doing?"

"Last night he stopped making any urine and was very puffy. I was worried his kidney function was shutting down. However, today he made a small amount of urine."

Aceline's mood perks up. "Thank God. Most patients who stop making urine end up dying. The fact that he is starting to urinate means he could be on his way to recovery. Have you seen Bonte?"

"Yes. I told Bonte that the HIV blood test on the patient is negative. He was relieved and immediately went back to work."

She high-fives David. "Finally, some good news."

***

The following day, David receives a call from Bokome, who until recently was the manager of one of the healthcare clinics in Kinshasa. Last month, he became the Director of the WHO office in Kinshasa after the previous Director was caught selling medical supplies on the black market. David had suspected that the supply shortage, including drugs, was due, at least in part, to corruption that is rampant in many of the countries he has worked in. When the shortage started to affect his medical center, he relayed his concerns to the WHO and an investigation found that the Director and another worker in the WHO office were selling some of the supplies to a criminal group. The WHO fired them both, but no arrests occurred. The WHO and UN have been fighting corruption for years with some success, but there is still a long battle ahead.

David likes Bokome, but knows he is on a steep learning curve trying to understand all the aspects of running the WHO office in Kinshasa. Bokome has some good news. "The supplies are ready and will be delivered to you tomorrow, but we still don't have additional healthcare workers to send your way."

David tries to contain his frustration but loses the battle. "This really pisses me off. If you can't even get us a small number of additional healthcare workers, how the hell are you going to find the hundreds of people needed to do a mass vaccination campaign in Kinshasa?"

"David, I am not an idiot. I called the WHO Headquarters in Geneva and they are working with the WHO African regional leadership to get us additional healthcare workers from other countries."

David shouts into the phone, "They better get here soon. I am fed up with all the excuses!" Bokome hangs up and David realizes that losing his cool will probably not help him get what they need, but it has at least temporarily reduced the intensity of his headache.

The WHO Regional African office sends additional healthcare workers to the Kuzi medical facility a few days later. These workers lessen the burden on those caring for patients, but the yellow fever outbreak has now spread into Kinshasa with over 20 people already hospitalized. The WHO Regional African office asks David and Aceline to start working on plans for a mass vaccination campaign that would include Kinshasa and surrounding areas. That night, Aceline and David begin planning, but they quickly realize that the available global supply of yellow fever vaccine is inadequate to complete the needed campaign. They proceed to develop a plan to use a reduced dose of the vaccine. David knows this plan needs the approval of Ann Leung, the WHO Director-General. David calls Maria Costa, the person he directly reports to in Geneva. Maria tells David she will arrange a time for him to talk with the Director-General, but it would be best if he meets with her in person rather than by phone.

Chapter 2

WHO Headquarters, Geneva, Switzerland, May 2016

Later that week, David takes a one-stop overnight flight from Kinshasa International Airport and arrives in Geneva at 10:30 a.m. the following day. The meeting with the Director-General is not until 2 p.m., so he decides to take the short train ride into the Cornavin railway station in the center of Geneva. From there he walks 10 minutes to the Simple Café, one of his favorite restaurants overlooking Lake Geneva, and orders lunch while sitting at an outside table. He enjoys watching the diverse array of people from different countries strolling along the walkways that surround this part of the lake.

During lunch, his thoughts wander to Aceline. The first time they met, her tall sleek build struck him along with her jet-black hair and sparkling blue eyes. Over time, he has come to admire her keen intellect and emotional stability even under intense pressure. He wonders again if she feels the same, but can't think of a good way to broach the subject. In the past, he has only been in a serious relationship with two other women and neither worked in the medical field. Each relationship lasted less than two years and he was surprised that the reasons why this was so were essentially the same — he was too wrapped up in his own world and often unaware of their thoughts and needs. In retrospect, they were probably right. He knew he was not in love with either of them and wondered if that was the real problem.

His thoughts are interrupted by his cell phone alarm buzzing, reminding him that his meeting with the Director-General will occur in an hour. He pays the bill and takes bus #8 for the 15-minute ride to the WHO headquarters. He continues to think about Aceline until the bus approaches the Palace of Nations where the UN has its European Headquarters. His thoughts quickly switch to what he needs to tell the Director-General about the plan to reduce the dose of the yellow fever vaccine in the DRC yellow fever outbreak.

The bus makes its final stop a few minutes later at the top of the Avenue Apia where the WHO campus lies. He quickly walks over to the building where his office is located to drop off his coat and then peeks next door into the office of Dr. Maria Costa, the Interim-Director of the WHO Emergency Division. Her secretary welcomes David back and tells him Maria is in a meeting, but will meet him at the waiting area outside the Director-General's office. David walks back to his office and writes a quick outline of the information he wants to convey to the Director-General. Maria and David catch up quickly before the administrative assistant invites them into the office.

The Director-General greets David. "I really appreciate you taking the time to travel here from the DRC on short notice. Maria has briefed me on the recent spread of the yellow fever outbreak into Kinshasa. Can you provide me with further details?"

"Sure. The current yellow fever outbreak in the DRC is already occurring in Angola and may now have crossed over to Uganda. Even more concerning is that the disease is now in Kinshasa and is rapidly spreading amongst the large population in the city. We are planning a mass vaccination campaign in Kinshasa and its surrounding areas. This will require about ten million doses of the vaccine. However, there are less than three million doses left in the central stockpile since 3.5 million doses were recently shipped to Brazil to deal with their worsening yellow fever outbreak."

"How many cases of yellow fever in Kinshasa have there been to date?"

"There are now 11 confirmed cases in Kinshasa and we are at a point where the cases are doubling every few days."

"This is very disturbing. Maria tells me that you are working on a plan that would allow the vaccination of everyone with a reduced dose of the vaccine. Has this ever been done before?"

"No, but there are several published studies done in volunteers that suggest we can use one-fifth of the normal vaccine dose and still get an immune response that will protect people from getting the disease."

The Director-General's voice expresses her level of concern. "I realize there might not be any other way to protect everyone at risk of getting yellow fever. However, if the reduced dose does not provide an adequate immune response, we will end up with millions of vaccinated, but unprotected people, against yellow fever. This could result in more deaths than if we did a smaller campaign with the full dose. Additionally, a mass vaccination campaign that does not protect the population from the disease could negatively impact all of the hard work we've done to get the people in the DRC to participate in regular vaccination programs."

"I understand the risks, but I am confident it will work."

The Director-General sits silently for a few minutes. She knows David is very good at his job, but can also be overconfident. Finally, she looks up at David and Maria. "Let's do this. I'll set up an emergency teleconference meeting of the WHO Strategic Advisory Committee of Experts (SAGE) on Immunizations to seek their input."

David knows that SAGE is the WHO's principal advisory group on issues related to the use of vaccines. He believes there is enough evidence to convince SAGE members to recommend the use of a reduced dose of yellow fever vaccine in this outbreak. "This sounds great. Do you think we can arrange the call within the next few days?"

"My office will work on finding the earliest possible date that most SAGE members are available."

"The sooner the better."

Maria thanks the Director-General for helping them expedite a potential solution for the yellow fever vaccine shortage. She walks back with David to her office without saying a word. Once there, she angrily tells David, "You should not have talked to the Director-General that way!"

David looks surprised. "What do you mean?"

"When she said she would set up the SAGE teleconference as quickly as possible, you responded by saying the sooner the better. You don't threaten the Director-General!"

"I wasn't trying to threaten her. I was conveying the urgency."

Maria is now furious. "Do you really think she doesn't understand the seriousness of the problem? David, you are very good at what you do, but at times you lack insight into how to deal with colleagues and can really make people angry, including me."

***

The following day David, Maria and other members of the WHO Emergency Division with expertise in yellow fever explore potential other options for increasing the yellow fever vaccine supply. Based on discussions with the four companies that make the yellow fever vaccine, there is very little manufacturing capacity to make additional vaccines in the short term. The group decides to focus their attention on the information that exists to determine the lowest dose that will still protect people.

Two days later, SAGE has the emergency teleconference to discuss whether using a reduced dose of the yellow fever vaccine is reasonable. SAGE is composed of 15 independent experts from around the globe that normally meet twice a year and provide the WHO with recommendations on the introduction and use of vaccines in developing countries. In exceptional emergency circumstances, such as the 2009 influenza pandemic, SAGE can hold unscheduled meetings and issue recommendations for consideration by the Director-General.

During the emergency call, SAGE members are updated on the increasing spread of yellow fever in the DRC. They then review the available evidence on the immune response of humans to lower doses of the yellow fever vaccine. SAGE members ask various clarifying questions and then discuss whether they think reducing the dose is reasonable. SAGE decides there is sufficient evidence to determine that one-fifth of the standard yellow fever vaccine dose should provide the number of doses needed for the mass campaign while protecting those vaccinated.

SAGE notes several issues requiring further consideration prior to starting this new campaign. A few years earlier, SAGE concluded there was sufficient evidence to indicate that the yellow fever vaccine offered life-long protection and recommended that everyone receiving the vaccine needed only one dose, rather than repeated doses every ten years as previously recommended. However, there is no evidence to determine if the reduced dose will provide life-long protection and studies are needed to answer this question. Therefore, SAGE recommends that those receiving the reduced vaccine dose be informed of this issue.

SAGE also expresses concern that despite having a very good vaccine that provides life-long protection at full dosage, various countries in Africa and South America are still experiencing repeated yellow fever outbreaks due to insufficient use of the vaccine. SAGE requests that a more comprehensive plan to eliminate yellow fever from these countries be developed and presented at their next regularly scheduled meeting.

***

The next morning Maria leaves for Brazil to get a better understanding of the extent of the yellow fever outbreak there and whether a reduced dose of vaccine will be required. David meets alone with the Director-General to update her on the SAGE recommendations. She tells him she supports the plan to use the reduced dose of the vaccine. David is about to leave the office when she asks him to stay to discuss another item.

"David, the 2014 Ebola outbreak in Western Africa and the current yellow fever outbreak in the DRC have convinced me that a new global approach is needed to deal more effectively with the increasing number of emergency situations occurring worldwide. Based on consultations with a number of outside experts, I have decided to combine the existing WHO departments that respond to various types of crises into a single Health Emergencies Program Division. The final components of this plan are still under consideration, but in the meantime, I need someone to be the Interim-Director of the Health Emergencies Program. I hope you will take on this role."

This request shocks David. He quickly regains his composure. "How far along is the planning process for this new program?"

"The idea has been percolating in my brain for over a year. The biggest issue we face dealing with emergencies is that most of the outside funding the WHO receives is designated for infectious disease outbreaks that affect high-income countries as well as developing countries. We are now developing a WHO Research and Development Blueprint to expedite the discovery of new medical products needed to deal with diseases mainly impacting low- and middle-income countries. Currently, these products take decades to develop and bring to market. This program aims to substantially decrease the time needed to develop and manufacture new products for these countries."

"Will this program have additional resources?"

"We are currently soliciting additional monies to support this program from the leadership of various countries and organizations. Our initial goal is to raise at least $500 million before the end of the year.

"Why are you asking me to be the Interim-Director, rather than Maria or other more senior WHO leadership?"

"David, you have a lot of experience dealing with disease outbreaks. You are also very innovative, as noted by your newest plan for dealing with the expanding yellow fever emergency. Furthermore, you know most of the internal WHO people and external partners that deal with emergencies on site. If you do a good job as Interim-Director, there is a good chance you will be made the permanent Director."

"Have you discussed this with other WHO leadership and outside partners and were they in favor of me taking this position?"

"Most were, but some expressed concerns that at times you are dismissive of the ideas of others. You will need to be more collaborative with the partners and listen to their concerns and suggestions, while still holding everyone accountable for fulfilling their roles. This will not be an easy job, but I am confident you are up to the task."

"Can I think about it and give you my answer tomorrow before I go back to the DRC."

"Okay, but I do hope you will say yes."

David decides that walking home will help him clear his head and goes back to his office to get his coat. During the hour walk home, he considers whether he can be successful in this new position, and how the position aligns with his career goals. He thought he stands a chance of taking over Maria's position when she retires in a few years, but this offer goes way beyond that next career step. His success will depend on being able to implement the WHO Research and Development Blueprint for infectious disease outbreaks, but also other causes of emergencies he has little experience with, including natural disasters such as flooding and those caused by armed conflicts. His modest experience dealing with outside groups that provide funding for disasters is another major concern.

The time flies by quickly and as he gets closer to home, his stomach is gnawing with hunger. He stops at the Ali Haydar Kebab restaurant to pick up a kebab sandwich. Upon arriving home, he sits in his lounge chair and devours the kebab. He quickly falls asleep in the chair, but a few hours later he wakes up and his mind continues to race with conflicting thoughts about whether he should take the job. As the sun rises, he finally decides to accept the position despite his many concerns. He cannot exactly pinpoint why he came to this conclusion, except he is convinced it will allow him to make a bigger difference in improving global health. He emails the Director-General his acceptance of the new position. He then calls Aceline and tells her that the Director-General has accepted their vaccine plan. He also asks if she can set up a meeting with Bokome at his office for the following day so that they can begin planning the vaccine campaign. She agrees to do this and offers to pick him up at the Kinshasa airport.

Chapter 3

Kinshasa, DRC
May to August 2016

David gives Aceline a warm hug when he sees her waiting for him at the airport. "I have some big news to tell you."

The hug surprises her since he has never done that before, but assumes he is just excited that their vaccine plan was approved. "I'm guessing your big news relates to some new aspect of the plan."

"Not really, but if we have time, I want to take you out for lunch and we can talk about it there."

"That should work since our meeting with Bokome is at 3 p.m. Where do you want to eat?"

"How about ASK Tabuinhas? On Sunday, they have a great lunch buffet."

"A hug and an offer to go to one of my favorite restaurants. This must be really good news."

At the restaurant, David asks for a table in a relatively private corner. They go to the buffet area and choose from a variety of foods that include Italian, French, Mediterranean, and Portuguese dishes. Once back at their table, they share the different foods they have chosen. Their favorite is the Portuguese bacalhau, a dish that has scrambled eggs filled with fried potatoes and cod. When they finish eating, Aceline looks at David. "Okay, enough stalling. Let me hear the big news."

"After the Director-General approved our plan, she told me she had something else we needed to discuss. She asked me to take on the role of Interim-Director of a new Health Emergencies Program she is creating."

"What did you say?"

"After thinking about it overnight, I accepted the position."

Aceline's face turns pale. "I'm shocked."

"Are you surprised because she asked me to take this position?"

Aceline realizes she is upset for both work and personal reasons, but right now needs to focus the conversation on the impact this will have on the yellow fever outbreak. "How can you possibly accept that position while we are in the midst of this expanding outbreak?"

"When I sent my acceptance email, I asked her to let me stay in the DRC until this outbreak is under control."

"What did she say?"

"She asked me to update her on how the vaccine campaign is impacting the outbreak on a regular basis, and together we will decide when it is time to assume the Interim-Director position."

"I don't understand why you want this position given the severe criticism the WHO received over how it handled the 2014 Ebola outbreak in Western Africa."

"Currently, the WHO is trying to deal with outbreaks and humanitarian crises in more than 40 countries. The Director-General has promised to redesign how the WHO responds to these disasters including the creation of this new Health Emergencies Program that works across all levels of the organization. She is currently in the process of meeting with various countries and funding organizations to raise the money for this program. She promised me the needed resources to do the job and felt confident I had the ability to help her get this done."

Aceline knows that she needs to calm down and decides to switch the subject. "David, let's continue this conversation later, right now we need to drive to the WHO Kinshasa office and meet with Bokome so that we can focus on the current issue at hand."

For the rest of the ride, David sits in silence, dismayed that Aceline does not seem happy about his promotion. Once they arrive at the office, David puts his disappointment aside and begins to highlight for Bokome and Aceline the SAGE conference call discussion and his conversation with the Director-General that will allow them to proceed with an expanded campaign using a reduced dose of the yellow fever vaccine.

He wraps up the overview by saying, "We will be giving most people one-fifth the normal dose even though the vaccine is only licensed to use at a full dose."

Bokome asks, "Do we need to create a consent form since we are using the reduced dose of the vaccine?"

"Great question and the answer is 'yes'. The consent form must clearly indicate we are using a reduced dose of the vaccine because the disease has now spread into Kinshasa. The form should note this is the only way we can protect everyone at risk and there is evidence to support that the reduced dose will protect people during the current outbreak. Additionally, we do need to note that it is currently unknown whether the reduced dose will provide the life-long protection that the full dose does."

Bokome inquires, "Will we do a research study during the campaign that will allow us to eventually answer this question?"

"Yes. We need several hundred people who have received the reduced vaccine to agree to let us obtain blood from them on two occasions: at the time we give them the vaccine, and a year later. It would be best if we can do this in a few easily accessible villages. Those agreeing to be in this study need to be given an additional consent form that will explain the purpose of the study is to determine if their yellow fever virus antibody levels after a year are similar to what we already know will happen with those given the full dose of the vaccine."

One of Bokome's staff asks, "Are there any groups we should be giving the full dose?"

"Another good question. SAGE highlighted the lack of data on reduced dosing in children less than two years of age and pregnant women, and recommended they be given the full dose."

Bokome raises another issue. "Some ethnic groups don't trust those who work with the DRC government. This may make it particularly difficult to explain to them why we want to vaccinate using a reduced vaccine dose. There is an anthropologist who works with different cultural groups in the DRC and she could be helpful."

Aceline thinks she knows the person Bokome is talking about. "I like your suggestion. Are you talking about Professor Kamanda Mutombo at the University of Kinshasa?"

"Yes. Do you know her?"

"I do. Kamanda has helped us on several occasions in work with marginalized populations in the DRC. She understands the reasons for their mistrust of the DRC government and outside organizations. Her ability to speak various dialects and her in-depth knowledge of the different concerns of these groups has enabled her to gain their trust. Most recently, when yellow fever cases started to occur in the Twa villages, she was able to convince the leaders the vaccine was safe and would protect them from getting the disease. I will contact her and see if she is available to help us."

David continues with the plan, "We need to continue our campaign in the rural areas, but start to use the reduced dose of vaccine. We also need to finish estimating the number of doses of vaccine we will need for those living in Kinshasa and its surrounding areas, and whether each health center in Kinshasa has enough working cold storage units for the vaccine vials that need to be kept there."

Bokome answers, "The last population census done in Kinshasa showed we had over ten million people living in the area. The census occurred several years ago, so it would be best if we increase this number to 11 million. I will check with the vaccine district manager regarding their storage capacity. Can we get more cold storage equipment if needed?"

David nods. "The Director-General assured me we could get all the supplies and equipment needed."

Aceline raises another matter. "We need to explain to our healthcare workers why a reduced dose of the vaccine will be used and how they can administer it."

Bokome responds, "We will ask all our district clinic managers to come to our office this week to learn about this. They can then disseminate the information to those they supervise."

David, Aceline and Bokome spend the rest of the afternoon and most of the evening doing detailed planning for the mass vaccination campaign and conclude that 2.5 million vaccine full doses should be sufficient to vaccinate everyone with a reduced dose of the vaccine and still have enough full doses left for young children and pregnant women. The following day, David and Aceline head back to their rural clinic.

***

Over the next week, Bokome works with his staff and managers to hire and train additional personnel to help with the campaign. He also receives and disperses the additional cold storage units needed by the various healthcare districts in Kinshasa. However, just as he is ready to call David to set a date to begin the mass campaign, he becomes aware of another problem.

Bokome calls David. "We finished training several hundred additional healthcare workers and are almost ready to start the vaccine campaign. However, my staff just informed me that foreign mining and construction workers from Kenya and China working in the DRC and Angola developed yellow fever upon returning to their home countries. Both countries are now reporting several cases of yellow fever in people who did not travel outside their own country."

This news does not surprise David. "I was worried this might happen since the same mosquitoes that transmit the yellow fever virus between people in the DRC are also present in other countries that have people working in the DRC. I had hoped the WHO International Health Regulations requirements for yellow fever vaccination certificates for travelers coming to the DRC and Angola would be enforced, so no foreigner could enter the DRC without proof they received the yellow fever vaccine."

Bokome agrees. "Unfortunately, these regulations are not fully enforced in the DRC. Some immigration officials can be bribed and a market in fake vaccination certificates has developed."

"Have you talked to Maria?"

"Right before I called you. She said they would talk with the health ministers in each of the relevant countries to make it clear no one can enter the DRC or Angola without documentation of yellow fever vaccination. In the meantime, Maria felt the best thing we could do at this point is start the mass campaign as soon as possible."

"I agree. I will ask Aceline to call you later today to confirm her group is ready."

***

Aceline and Bokome arrange to meet the next day and have asked Kamanda Mutombo to join them. Aceline spoke with Kamanda the week before and she agreed to help them communicate with various ethnic groups regarding why a reduced vaccine dose is necessary.

Aceline arrives at the WHO Kinshasa office around 7 a.m. and Bokome and Kamanda are already there. Aceline greets Kamanda warmly. "Kamanda, I can't thank you enough for the help you have already provided and for taking the time to meet with us today."

Kamanda smiles. "I am honored to be part of the work you are doing. This yellow fever outbreak has been the worst one I can remember and I am grateful for the help you are giving to my people."

"Kamanda, the work you have already done to create different consent forms for specific ethnic groups will allow us to move up the vaccination campaign starting date. The most pressing problem right now is creating a consent form for pregnant women and another form for families with children less than two years of age."

"Just before you arrived today, Bokome told me children under two years of age would receive a full dose of the vaccine because there is no data on whether a reduced dose will work in them. I can incorporate that information into the final consent forms. However, I need to better understand why you are also singling pregnant women out for a full dose?"

Aceline explains, "Pregnant women are at greater risk of death compared to women of a similar age who are not pregnant. Additionally, the chance of her unborn child surviving is very small even if the baby is approaching 40 weeks gestation. Furthermore, if the mother has other young children, the chance of them surviving to five years of age without her, is around 10% in low-income countries such as the DRC."

"Is this increased risk of death in pregnant women true only for yellow fever?"

"Actually, there are other viruses that also cause higher mortality in pregnant women and their fetuses, including Ebola, influenza and hepatitis E."

"Is this true only for viruses?"

"Unfortunately, not. For instance, the bacteria that cause cholera and the parasite that causes malaria both result in increased mortality in pregnant women."

"Is this increased risk of death why pregnant women are getting a full dose of the yellow fever vaccine?"

"One of several reasons. The yellow fever vaccine contains a live attenuated yellow fever virus strain grown in cells cultures."

"What do you mean by attenuated?" Kamanda asks.

"The vaccine strain is passed through the cells multiple times so that it is weakened enough that it does not cause disease in people, but yet induce an immune response."

"If the virus is attenuated, why were pregnant women not given the vaccine previously?"

"In the past, pregnant women were excluded from receiving the yellow fever vaccine, or any other live virus vaccine, because of concerns that even though the virus in the vaccine was weakened, it might cause harm to the unborn child. Several years ago, SAGE recommended vaccinating pregnant women during yellow fever outbreaks after considering the high mortality risk in the mother and baby and the excellent safety record of the vaccine."

"How do they know the vaccine is safe if pregnant women never got the vaccine?"

"Kamanda, you are asking really good questions. Over 500 million doses of the yellow fever vaccine have been given to people over many years and during this time a substantial number of women who did not realize they were pregnant inadvertently received the vaccine. Despite this, there have not been any reports of pregnant women getting yellow fever from the vaccine itself."

"So why did SAGE recommend that pregnant women get the full dose of the vaccine rather than the reduced dose?"

"The previous SAGE recommendation to use the yellow fever vaccine in pregnant women was based on using a full dose of the vaccine. When SAGE recommended using the reduced dose of the vaccine a few weeks ago, they specifically noted pregnant women should get a full dose because their immune response might be different than those who are not pregnant."

Kamanda considers what Aceline has told her and comes to a decision. "In order to come up with a good communication plan, it is important I talk with pregnant women in a few villages to understand how they feel about getting the vaccine, particularly since it is a different dose from what others in their family will get. This will help us create communications that directly address their issues."

"How long do you think this will take?"

"A few days."

***

During the next few months, millions of people in Kinshasa and its surrounding areas receive the yellow fever vaccine. The number of yellow fever cases is declining and everyone feels the campaign is going well. David and Aceline have arrived in the WHO's office in Kinshasa to work with Bokome on a long-term vaccine plan to stop these recurring outbreaks.

David puts several papers on the table where they will work on the plan. "Yesterday, I called Maria to update her on the status of the vaccination campaign and informed her we are seeing a substantial decrease in the number of patients seeking care. I told her that with Kamanda's help, very few people were refusing the vaccine and the biggest problem was that the large lines of people at some of the vaccination sites were causing long waiting times. She then told me about a new plan SAGE was considering that would incorporate using the yellow fever vaccine into the routine childhood vaccination program. She believes this plan can substantially decrease the number of yellow fever outbreaks and sent me a draft of the proposed plan. She asked me to consider whether we could put this plan into place in the DRC."

Bokome asks, "I heard SAGE's plan recommends giving one dose of the vaccine to infants at one year of age. Are you sure one dose will provide long-term protection and stop these recurring yellow fever outbreaks from occurring?"

"Spraying insecticides and providing bed nets in villages to stop the mosquito-borne diseases has been ongoing for decades. While these interventions help decrease the incidence of malaria, yellow fever, and other mosquito-transmitted diseases to some degree, the mosquitoes are, over time, becoming resistant to the spray and are biting more in the daytime. Thus, SAGE felt other interventions are needed and after over seven decades of using the vaccine in various countries, they felt there was substantial evidence that the protection from the vaccine lasts for many decades and likely a lifetime."

"Donors are paying for the current campaign. Who is going to pay for the routine use of the vaccine in infants?"

"Maria said the Director-General has already talked to the DRC Prime Minister who promises to find the money to pay for the vaccine given to infants."

Aceline scoffs. "I'll believe it when I see it. However, right now we can work with the DRC Health Minister and provide him with any help he needs."

"Maria asked me to tell you that the Director-General really appreciates the work we have done. Now she wants me to travel to Brazil to help her deal with an outbreak of Zika virus that appears to be causing congenital abnormalities in the fetuses of pregnant women."

"Oh wow. How soon are you leaving?" Aceline asks.

"In three days."

Later that day, David and Aceline drive back to the medical facility in Kuzi. Aceline is unusually quiet and David suspects she is thinking about what his leaving will mean.

"Aceline, I meant to tell you when we were driving to Kinshasa that I would be leaving in a few days. I am comfortable we are finally getting the outbreak under control and I'm confident that Bokome and you will do a great job of finishing the task."

"I don't doubt we can do that."

"Then what's bothering you?"

Aceline stares at him. "Are you really so focused on work that nothing else enters your brain?"

David thinks for a moment and despite his uncertainty, decides to raise the question about the nature of their relationship. "Are you talking about us?"

"Well, yes. Do you ever think that you and I could be something more than friends?"

"I've thought about it frequently, but I couldn't tell if you were interested."

Aceline is now more upset. "So now that you are leaving in three days, we are finally going to broach this topic? Why didn't you ever say anything?"

David thinks for a second and then responds. "Why didn't you ever say anything?"

Aceline reluctantly cracks a smile even though she is irritated. "Ugh, that's an annoyingly good point. I don't know if I should laugh or cry."

"How about be happy? I would very much like to see if we could make it work."

"Ha. I don't think three days will do the trick."

"Maria thought I wouldn't need to be in Brazil for more than a week. Once I am back, I will see what I can arrange so you and I can spend some time together away from work. Do you have any vacation time you can take?"

"I'm owed a lot of vacation time."

"Let's both think about where we want to go. Wherever that is, I would love to spend time with you away from work."

Aceline takes David's hand, "I look forward to it."

Chapter 4

Sao Paulo, Brazil, September 2016

David's flight from Kinshasa to Sao Paulo, Brazil, involves three separate flights and takes over 24 hours. He arrives on Tuesday, September 6, 2016, in the late afternoon and takes a taxi to the Ibis Styles São Paulo Centro Hotel where a room has been booked for him. He calls room service to order dinner and then finishes reading the background information that Maria sent him.

David soon realizes his knowledge of the Zika virus is rudimentary — he only knows that the virus infects humans through the bite of the *Aedes* species of mosquitoes, but rarely causes serious disease. He originally thought Africa and Asia were the only regions where the virus lived, but now learns that the virus invaded Brazil in 2015. By 2016, the virus had spread to 26 countries and territories in the Americas. Most people infected with the virus are asymptomatic. Those who do become ill, generally have mild to moderate signs and symptoms, including a fever, rash, joint pain and conjunctivitis. Deaths from Zika virus infection are rare in persons of all ages.

The next day, David has a series of meetings with public health officials and begins to understand what is so different about the outbreak in Brazil. The recent introduction of the virus into Brazil where no one was previously exposed to the virus meant that everyone was susceptible to infection by mosquitoes carrying the virus. This resulted in large numbers of infected people over a short time period. There is also a marked increase in the number of reports of infants with very small heads being born to pregnant women. The term for this condition is microcephaly, and it was severe enough for parents to notice and become upset upon first seeing their newborn infants. Other findings detected in some infants include abnormalities of the eye, central nervous system, and skeleton.

David's last meeting of the day is with Pedro Oliveira, who is the Director of Epidemiology in the Sao Paulo Public Health Division. He has over 20 years of experience examining the incidence and distribution of various diseases, and other factors that affect public health. During the last year, he has led the government's effort in tracking the spread of the Zika virus within Brazil. He shows David a map highlighting where all the suspected cases of newborn microcephaly have occurred.

"Pedro, the map seems to suggest that in some towns and cities in Brazil, there is a large number of microcephaly cases by the virus while other places have not had a single case."

"You may be right. Initially, I thought this was just a reporting artifact due to some places not having the capacity to detect and/or report cases. However, this past month, I visited some of the areas that have not reported any cases and looked at the records of infants born there during the last year. Based on my initial review, I could not find any missed cases. Next week, some members of my team will be going to these areas to see if the mosquitoes in these places contain the virus."

David and Pedro continue to talk for another 45 minutes. When the meeting finishes at 4:30 p.m., he asks Pedro whether he knows someone who is caring for affected newborns. Pedro suggests he meet with Dr. Venetia Sousa, a friend of his who cares for infants and does research on the virus. Pedro calls her and she agrees to meet David in the main lobby of the Sao Paulo Medical Center at 6 p.m. Pedro offers to drive David over to the medical center, but David insists it will not be a problem for him to take a taxi. He arrives at the medical center lobby a few minutes early and thinks he sees her sitting in the lobby, a tall pregnant woman with brown hair.

He walks over to the woman and asks, "Are you Dr. Sousa?"

"Yes, please call me Venetia. Pedro said the WHO sent you here to learn more about the Zika virus outbreak. Can you tell me a little about yourself and what you're trying to learn?"

"Hi, my name is David Ferguson and my friends call me David. During the past two years, I have been in the DRC caring for patients affected by the yellow fever outbreak. I also oversaw the yellow fever vaccination campaign. Last week, the WHO Director-General asked me to take on the position of Interim-Director of the WHO Health Emergencies Program. The Director-General asked me to come to Brazil to see how the WHO could help with the Zika virus outbreak. Today, I met with various public health officials who have given me a detailed update on the extent of the outbreak. They suggested that I meet with you since you provide care for infants infected by the Zika virus and also work with the Pan American Health Organization on research projects related to the outbreak."

"David, it is nice to meet you. We certainly welcome any assistance the WHO can provide. Perhaps the first thing we should do is go into the nursery where there are currently two infants born to mothers who were infected with the Zika virus during their pregnancy."

They take an elevator up to the sterile-looking nursery and Venetia takes David over to a bassinette where one of the Zika infected infants is lying. "The mom of this baby was infected with the Zika virus. The mom never had any symptoms, but an ultrasound done while she was in her third trimester suggested that the baby had microcephaly. The Zika antibody tests showed that the mom had most likely been infected in her first or second trimester."

David looks at the infant. "I can see that head is small. Do you know what the head circumference percentile is?"

"Well below the third percentile. The baby was born late this morning and we have a CT scan of the head scheduled for tomorrow to get a better feel for the actual size of the brain and whether there are any abnormal areas in the brain."

"Are there any other physical indications of Zika on this infant?"

"Not that we can see, but the other infant we have in the nursery has multiple other findings."

They walk across the nursery to where the other infant is. "The mother of this baby had symptoms of fever and fatigue for several days during the first trimester. Antibody testing confirmed that she had the Zika virus. Based on serial ultrasounds done during her pregnancy, we knew the baby had developed microcephaly. The baby was born two days ago and there were other indications of Zika, including scarring in the back of the eye, increased muscle tone, and clubfoot."

David gets Venetia's permission to examine the baby and goes over to the sink to wash his hands before touching the infant. He notices how small the head is and the shape of the skull appears asymmetric. He notes the right clubfoot and the infant's legs feel tight when he moves them. "I read about some of these physical exam findings, but seeing them up close is more troubling than I thought. How are the mothers doing?"

"Both sets of parents are very concerned and are asking questions about how their infants will do going forward. It is hard to know what to tell them since we have been following infants affected by the virus for less than a year. What we have seen to date is that infants with microcephaly appear to be developmentally delayed."

Venetia looks away and wipes a tear from her eye. "The parents have a very hard time dealing with what we tell them and the uncertainty makes it worse."

David decides it is time to move to another topic. "Is it okay if we change the conversation to your research projects?"

"Sure, what would you like to hear about?"

"Tell me about the research projects you are involved with."

"Of course. I am part of two research projects. The first study uses mosquitoes that were genetically altered in a laboratory so that they can't reproduce. We are introducing the altered mosquito into a few neighborhoods to determine if this will lead to an overall reduction of mosquitoes in the area. To date, we demonstrated a 25% reduction in the number of mosquitoes, and are now trying to determine if this will result in a decrease in the incidence of people infected with the virus."

"That's great initial data. I know other researchers are trying something similar in Africa to see if they can decrease the number of cases of malaria. You said you were also working on another project. Can you tell me about that?"

"The US National Institutes of Health has provided grant support to various research groups who are trying to develop a vaccine to prevent Zika virus infections. They have already done some studies in primates and a Phase 1 study involving a small number of healthy non-pregnant adult volunteers. One of the vaccines appears to produce a good immune response and our research group has been asked to start planning for a Phase 2 study that will examine the safety and efficacy of the vaccine in a larger number of patients."

"It would be great if I could hear more details about these studies. Are you available to continue this conversation over dinner?"

"That sounds good. Let me call my fiancé, Luiz, and tell him I will be home later than usual."

After talking with Luiz, she suggests they go to a restaurant down the street that is quite good. They walk for a few minutes and arrive at the restaurant. At Venetia's request, the maître-de sits them at a corner table.

"Venetia, what would you suggest I order?"

"This restaurant is renowned for its churrascaria (barbecued meats) that are served on skewers. I am particularly fond of the lamb, but they also have really good pork and wild boar barbecue."

Venetia orders the lamb and a glass of sparkling water for herself. For David, she orders the pork along with a glass of Salton Paradoxo Pinot Noir. David then asks Venetia what made her decide to become a physician and researcher.

"My career choices starts back when I was a child. I grew up in a very poor Catholic family living in *Barrio de La Boca in Sao Paulo*, which is a favela."

"Can you explain to me what a favela is?"

"A favela is a slum area of which, unfortunately, there are many in Brazil. You probably noticed the one close to the hospital as you were walking over. My parents worked very hard to provide for our family and were constantly encouraging me to do well in school so that I could find a career that would allow me a better life. After graduating from high school, I was able to get a scholarship to attend the University of Sao Paulo and study Life Sciences. After graduating, I decided to attend the Sao Paulo Medical School since it allowed me to achieve some of my most important goals, including helping my family get out of the favela and providing care for those who still live there."

"What did you do after finishing medical school?"

"I did a pediatric residency and then worked at a clinic in my hometown for four years. I enjoyed caring for children, but decided that in order to help improve the health of impoverished children on a larger scale, I needed more training in public health. I went back to the University of Sao Paulo to get a Master's degree in public health and, during that time, I participated in several research studies with one of my professors. The research involved designing and implementing health education programs in favelas for families to empower them to provide better health for themselves. My mentor thought I was doing a good job and convinced the Medical School to offer me a position on the faculty.

"Currently, I provide pediatric care for two half-days per week at the medical center and I spend the rest of my time doing research. I have been overseeing the mosquito study in a town just outside of Sao Paulo for over a year. Recently, the leader of the National Institute of Allergy and Immunology asked the Director of the Pan American Health Organization research section to begin planning for a Zika vaccine trial in Brazil, and they asked me to be part of the planning group for the vaccine study."

"You said you were engaged. Is your fiancé also in medicine?"

"No. I met my fiancé, Luiz Moreno, three years ago at a fund-raising event for the Sao Paulo Medical Center. Luiz started his own information technology consultancy business about a decade ago and was at the event because he had previously donated money to the University. We dated off and on for a while, but this year our relationship became more serious and six months ago he proposed to me. We plan to get married next month and the baby is due in four months. Luiz is very excited that he will soon be a father."

"Are you excited?"

"Yes, but I am worried about the Zika outbreak."

"Have you had an illness compatible with the Zika virus?"

"No, but most people who are infected with the virus don't develop any symptoms and recent data suggest infection of the fetus can occur any time during pregnancy. Next week I am seeing my Ob-Gyn and will ask her to do a blood test on me to see if I have evidence of being infected by the virus."

"I'm sure everything will be fine."

Venetia thinks his response is dismissive of her concerns and decides to move the discussion back to the research studies. "David, what else can I tell you about the proposed studies that would be helpful?"

"My expertise relates more to the vaccine study you are undertaking. However, I know a number of people at the WHO who are working to decrease the ability of mosquitoes to transmit diseases. Would it be helpful if one of them contacted you?"

"Yes. I'm particularly interested in what techniques they are using to quantify the impact of their interventions on the mosquito population and also the incidence of disease."

"I will talk with the mosquito research group as soon as I am back in Geneva. As for as the vaccine study, can you tell me what you know about the various vaccines that they are trying to develop, particularly the one they hope to use in the study you are planning?"

"I'm honestly not sure. I can ask that question when I am at the Pan American Health Organization office next week."

"Okay. Can you give me a brief overview of the planned study?"

"Sure. We already confirmed that the first part of this study should include women who are of childbearing age, but not pregnant and willing to use contraceptives to reduce the risk of pregnancy while in the study. I will be meeting with various Pan American Health Organization staff next week to discuss the number of people they need for the Phase 2 study and what laboratory work and outcomes we should follow. This meeting will be in the Pan American Health Organization office in San Paulo. Would you like to join us?"

"That would be great."

"It's getting late and I should get on home."

"I should too; it's been a long day."

The waiter brings the credit card machine over to their table and David pays for the meal. Venetia stands up and puts on her jacket. "I really appreciate you taking me to dinner. I will get back to you with a date and time for the meeting at the Pan American Health Organization office."

***

The restaurant is near where Venetia and Luiz live and she decides to walk home. She is glad the WHO is interested in helping with the Zika virus outbreak since this should speed up the process of understanding why some Zika virus-infected pregnant women have infants impacted by the disease. She has been concerned about this because early estimates of the percentage of affected infants range from 5% to 50% and there is a great need to know the actual number.

As a researcher, she knows she needs to stay objective, but as an expectant mother, she is very worried. David's comment that "everything will be fine" makes her realize that Luiz has the same feeling, but for different reasons. Luiz has a deep religious faith that gets him through troubled times, whether they relate to business, family or friends. This is one of his attributes that she admires most. However, she realizes they never really talked about the risk of the Zika virus infecting their child, nor has she expressed her concerns to him.

By the time she arrives home, she decides they need to have this conversation. Luiz is sitting in the living room when Venetia walks in.

"*Olá meu amor*. How are you?"

"Mostly good. David Ferguson is the head of the WHO Emergency Division and I think he can help us get the additional funding and expertise needed to speed up the research needed to understand how to deal with this Zika virus outbreak. In fact, he will be joining me in the Pan American Health Organization office meeting next week to discuss the design of the vaccine study."

"Wonderful. However, what did you mean by 'mostly good'? Is there something bothering you?"

She looks directly into Luiz's round smiling face and dark brown eyes and sees the boundless optimism that makes him so easy to love. She hopes this discussion will not alter his mood. "When I told David I was pregnant, he asked me if I was worried about whether our child could be infected with Zika virus."

"Are you worried about it?"

"Yes, and I realized I should have talked with you about my concerns before now."

"Well let's talk now. Why would he ask you that? You haven't had any illness since you became pregnant."

"Most people infected with Zika virus don't have any symptoms, which is a problem. Regardless of whether a pregnant woman has symptoms or not, the unborn babies can still be infected."

She notices his smile has disappeared and his forehead creases are showing. "How is that possible?"

"When a mosquito that contains the virus bites a person, the virus enters the bloodstream. Approximately 80% of the people infected with the virus have minimal or no symptoms, but the virus can infect the baby via the mom's blood."

"I had no idea. How often are babies affected?"

"We are not sure yet, but the most recent data suggests somewhere around 10% of women who get infected with the virus during pregnancy have affected babies."

"What happens to the baby if he or she gets infected?"

"The main problem we know of at this point is that the virus can cause the brain to develop abnormally."

"What do you mean?"

"Some of these children are being born with microcephaly, which means that their heads are small due to their brains not developing normally."

"What does that mean for the children in the long run?"

"Many of the infants are not reaching their normal physical and mental developmental milestones. There are also other problems that can happen. Abnormalities can also occur in their eyes and muscles. Some of these problems can be detected at birth, but others are noted during the first year."

Luiz looks very worried. "Are there tests that can be done to see if you have been infected with the Zika virus?"

"There is a blood test that looks at whether someone has developed antibodies to the Zika virus. However, this test has problems differentiating between the antibodies produced against the Zika and dengue viruses. Since both these viruses cause infections in Brazil, a positive test will not be definitive. If the test is negative, then we will know I have not been infected yet."

"You're five months pregnant. If you become infected between now and when the baby is born, is there still a risk our child could still be infected by the virus?"

"Unfortunately, yes. The virus can infect the baby anytime during the pregnancy."

Luiz sits and stares into space for a few minutes. He then moves closer to Venetia on the couch, holds her hand, and looks at her with tears streaming down his face. "I love you and we will deal with whatever happens. Your appointment with your Ob-Gyn is next week, so I'm going to cancel my business trip to Mexico and come with you."

She hugs him and he feels her tears dripping down his collar. "Luiz, I was worried what sharing this burden with you would do to our relationship, but I can tell it will bring us even closer together. I love you."

***

The following week Luiz goes with Venetia to the office of Dr. Mariana Santos, an obstetrician on the Sao Paulo Medical School faculty, and they discuss their concerns about whether their baby might have the Zika virus. The doctor agrees to send the blood test and schedule an ultrasound test to see if the baby is developing normally.

Luiz asks, "Would you normally be ordering an ultrasound test now?"

"We routinely do an ultrasound towards the end of the first trimester and when we did this for Venetia, everything looked good. I usually recommend getting additional ultrasounds in the second and third trimesters. Since Venetia is five months pregnant, we would normally get the second trimester ultrasound around this time."

"Will the ultrasound be able to tell if the baby will be born with abnormalities?"

"We should have the results from both tests within a week. The ultrasound can help us determine is if the head is growing normally, but can't rule out that the baby is infected."

"Why is that?"

"Some babies infected with Zika virus don't have small heads at birth, but can develop this or other problems over the first year after birth. I understand both of you are worried and the best thing we can do is get these tests done. When the test results are back, my office will set up another appointment for us to talk. In the meantime, I want to emphasize that even during this outbreak most women have normal babies."

Venetia wanted to let Luiz ask Dr. Santos any questions he had. He seemed to be okay with the answers for now. "Let's do the tests and then we can talk further once we know the results."

***

The next day David and Venetia meet at the Pan American Health Organization office, which is in the middle of downtown Sao Paolo, where several research staff members are working on plans for the Phase 2 study of the Zika virus vaccine. Venetia introduces David to the staff, and briefly shares his background and that the WHO has sent him to help them with the Zika virus outbreak.

David thanks them for letting him attend their planning session and sharing their study plans. The staff members provide David with an overview of the study plan and he then starts to ask questions. "What can you tell me about the vaccine?"

Carlos Rachinhas, the lead investigator on this study, answers. "Initially, the WHO hoped they could use a vaccine containing an inactivated Zika virus since a live virus vaccine in pregnant women could potentially cause congenital anomalies in the fetus even though the virus in the vaccine has been weakened. However, animal studies with the inactivated vaccine suggest that this type of vaccine may not be effective because it elicited a poor immune response.

"Multiple research groups have been working on developing other types of vaccines, and to date, the best vaccine appears to be a genetically engineered vector vaccine. The initial studies with this vaccine in animals produced a good immune response. A Phase 1 study involving 45 volunteers showed that the vaccine elicits an immune response to this Zika virus protein and did not reveal any serious side effects. The Phase 2 study needs to include about 500 participants to further examine if this vaccine is safe and to get a better indication of how good the immune response is. If this study indicates that the vaccine continues to look promising, then we will need to do a Phase 3 vaccine study in thousands of people."

Venetia looks puzzled. "Can you tell me what a vector vaccine is?"

Carlos knows the concept of a vector vaccine is new and not easy to grasp, particularly since none of the routinely recommended vaccines use this technology. "Vector vaccines use the replicative machinery of one virus to express one or more proteins from another virus that is causing the disease. For this vector Zika vaccine, they used two RNA viruses that are part of the Flavivirus family. A piece of the genetic material from the Zika virus that encodes the Zika virus protein they want to make an immune response to is incorporated into a weakened dengue virus that replicates in the hosts cells."

Venetia wants to make sure she understands the concept. "If I understand what you are saying, the live dengue virus is weakened so it does not cause disease in humans, but is still able to replicate in the cells of the person who is vaccinated. When the vaccine is injected into a person, the dengue virus replicates itself while also producing the Zika virus protein made from the genetic material inserted into the dengue virus genetic code."

"That is correct."

"Are there other viruses in the Flavivirus family that cause disease in humans?"

"There are about 70 viruses in the Flavivirus family. Approximately half of them cause disease in humans, but most don't cause large outbreaks. However, as David knows, yellow fever virus is another Flavivirus that causes widespread disease."

David does not want Venetia to feel like she should have known what a vector vaccine is. "I'd never heard of vector vaccines until two years ago when I was involved in the Ebola virus vector vaccine research study during the 2014 Ebola outbreak in Western Africa. It took me a while to understand this concept when I first heard it."

David asks another question. "Will this Phase 2 study include both men and women, and will pregnant women be included?"

"We plan to include women of childbearing age who are not pregnant. We are also thinking about including men because Venetia has shown us preliminary evidence suggesting Zika-virus-infected men can transmit the virus to women during intercourse."

"What is the evidence that sexual intercourse can lead to a woman being infected?"

Venetia responds to this question. "Zika virus infection occurred in some pregnant women who never lived in, or traveled to, an area with Zika virus. In most of these cases, their spouse had traveled to a Zika virus area during their pregnancy."

"Do they know how the virus is transmitted from a man to a woman?"

"The virus has been detected in the semen of infected men and can persist there for months."

The planning session goes on for several hours and David is impressed with the study design. Before leaving the Pan American Health Organization office, he promises the staff he will work with the WHO leadership to get them any additional help, including funding and additional expertise that is needed to complete this study.

***

A few days later, Venetia and Luiz return to the doctor's office to get the blood and ultrasound test results. Dr. Santos greets them and mentions that the second ultrasound test can determine whether the baby is a boy or girl.

"Would you like to know if your child is a girl or a boy?"

Venetia and Luiz had previously discussed this issue and agreed they would like to know the sex of their baby.

"You are the parents of a baby boy."

Venetia and Luiz smile at each other. Venetia follows up, "That's great. We've been very anxious while awaiting the results of the ultrasound and blood tests. What are the results?"

"The good news is the ultrasound does not show any signs of microcephaly. The blood test did come back positive, but blood tests can't tell the difference between someone infected with Zika, dengue or chikungunya viruses. The Aedes species of mosquitoes present in Brazil can transmit any of these viruses and each of these viruses can cause asymptomatic infections in people."

Luiz is puzzled. "I knew the test could not differentiate between Zika and dengue virus but hadn't heard about this chikungunya virus. What symptoms does the chikungunya virus cause? Can it cause abnormalities in the babies before they are born?"

"The main problem chikungunya causes is swelling and pain in the joints. Congenital infections, if they occur at all, are rare. Many people living in Brazil have experienced dengue virus infections and there is a good chance the positive test may be due to that virus."

They talk with Dr. Santos about what she plans for their next visit in a month. Upon leaving the doctor's office, they decide to have lunch at a nearby cafe. They sit at a table on the patio and order two salads with chicken. Luiz, ever the optimist, starts the conversation about what they learned at the doctor's office. "I understand we can't be certain whether our son has been infected with the Zika virus, but given the normal ultrasound results, I am hopeful he will be fine."

"So am I."

"What can we do to make sure you don't get infected by the Zika virus during the remaining months of the pregnancy?"

"Actually, we need to worry that neither of us gets infected since the male can be asymptomatic but carry the virus in his semen."

"You're right. I guess the best thing would be to avoid mosquitoes."

"We can't stay inside all day, but can use mosquito repellant".

"Are Aedes mosquitoes the only ones we need to worry about?"

"Anopheles mosquitoes are another species of mosquitoes found in Brazil and they transmit malaria. However, in Brazil, malaria rarely occurs outside the Amazon region. Since we will not be traveling to the Amazon area, at least while I am pregnant, this is not a problem."

"Are mosquito repellants safe for pregnant women?"

"There are certain types that are safe for pregnant women and we can also avoid going near areas of water where mosquitoes tend to hang out. This will reduce, but does not eliminate, the risk of mosquito bites. This is going to be tough because I seem to attract mosquitoes."

"What do you mean?"

"Mosquitoes are attracted to certain smells some people give off. When I sit outside, the mosquitoes seem to like to hang out around me rather than other people."

"Has no one come up with ways to kill these mosquitoes?"

"Research teams have been trying for many decades with only modest success. Insecticides have been developed that can kill mosquitoes, but mosquitoes can develop resistance to insecticides over time. This is exactly the reason I am doing research with genetically altered mosquitoes. The genetic changes do not kill the mosquito but stop them from being able to reproduce. Eventually, if they can't reproduce, the number of these mosquitoes should dramatically decrease."

"I am glad that someone as smart as you is doing this type of research. Is there anything else we can do now? I know in certain countries some people sleep under nets."

"These nets are now used mainly in areas of Africa where malaria is present. The netting contains insecticides and protects people sleeping in housing without window or door screens. However, the mosquitoes have developed behaviors that help them overcome the protection afforded by nets. For instance, mosquitoes tend to bite more at dusk and dawn, but in places that use the nets, these mosquitoes are biting more often in the daytime."

"Mosquitoes seem to be intelligent little buggers."

Venetia laughs. "If you think about it, the mosquitoes, like other species, adapt to survive."

"Let's talk about something more fun. Do you want to discuss names for our boy? Do you have a name in mind?"

"I have thought about boy and girl names on many occasions."

"I have a name for a boy. What do you think of Julio Rafael, which denotes that he is loved and wise?" says Luiz excitedly.

"I like the name. Tonight, when I'm sleeping, I will dream about our little Julio Rafael."

***

After attending a second research meeting at the Pan American Health Organization headquarters and talking with additional public health officials dealing with the Zika virus outbreak, David decides he is ready to head back to Geneva and meet with the Director-General about his findings. He sends an email to set up a meeting time, but learns the Director-General is away for a week.

David had been thinking a lot about where and when Aceline and he could go for a vacation. He decides that this is a great time to make that happen. He calls Aceline on her cell phone to find out if she is available.

"Aceline, I have been thinking about you a lot since I left for Brazil. How are you?"

"I'm glad to hear I am on your mind. I am doing okay. How has Brazil been?"

"Really interesting. I'm excited to share with you what I've learned. I didn't call to talk about my trip though. The Director-General is on vacation for the week, so I was wondering if you can take time off now?"

"Actually, yes. We finally have a full staff at the hospital. When and where do you propose we meet?"

"Depending on where we decide to go, I can meet you any place you want as early as tomorrow or the next day. I'm hoping we can spend a full week together."

"The yellow fever campaign is going fairly well and I think it is reasonable to take a vacation now. Let me talk with Bokome and see if he feels comfortable with me going away for a week. Are you still in Brazil?"

"Yes, but I've wrapped up my visit and don't have to be back in Geneva until I meet with the Director-General in ten days to report on the Zika virus outbreak."

"What do you think about meeting in Morocco? I think it's about halfway between Brazil and the DRC?"

"Works for me. Let me know what Bokome says."

Aceline calls David back that evening and tells him Bokome was fine with her taking a week off. She suggests they meet in two days at the Kenzi Tower Hotel in Casablanca. David wonders if he should ask if she wants him to make the hotel reservations, but doesn't feel comfortable broaching the subject of whether he should book one or two rooms. He decides he will get one room with a king-size bed and see when she gets there if she has booked her own room.

Chapter 5

Casablanca, Morocco
mid-October 2016

David arrives at the Kenzi Tower Hotel in the mid-afternoon. Aceline should arrive in the early evening and he goes to his room to shower and take a nap. He goes down to the lobby at 7 p.m. to wait for her to arrive. The hotel is a five-star luxury hotel and as he looks around in the lobby, he finds it a bit too extravagant for his taste. Most of the people coming in and out of the hotel are dressed in tuxedos and evening gowns. David has never been to Casablanca, and while he realizes it is a popular vacation spot, he wonders why Aceline chose this city and hotel for their vacation.

He orders a glass of chardonnay, but before the server returns, Aceline walks into the hotel. David is caught off guard because he initially did not recognize her. He always found her attractive, but at this moment he is struck by how truly beautiful she is. Previously, they had spent all their time together in rural Africa where their clothes were loose fitting and practical. Aceline is wearing a blue skirt and white blouse that highlights her figure that is both sleek and curvy. He comes over to her and, without thinking, hugs her tightly. He is delighted when she responds similarly. As he pulls away, he says, "I'm so glad to see you. How was your trip?"

"We hit a fair amount of turbulence while flying. I'm happy to be on the ground and here with you."

"I thought you might be tired, so I made an 8 p.m. dinner reservation at the hotel's restaurant on the 27th floor. I checked it out earlier; it has a great view of the city. Does that work for you?"

"That should be fine. Let me go check-in and freshen up and then I will meet you in the lobby."

"Do you want me to help you with your luggage?"

"The bellboys can bring it up."

A few minutes later, the server brings David the wine he ordered. He is trying to process several things that just happened. Based on her expression when she first saw him and her embrace, he believes she is happy to see him. She reserved her own hotel room, so he is glad he did not ask her whether he should make the hotel reservations. Based on his two previous relationships, he knows that his ability to read what the other person is thinking is not great, and wonders how he will know when she is ready to move their relationship forward. When he looks up, Aceline is standing in front of him.

"David, you seem deep in thought. Was it about work or us?"

"Perhaps we should talk about both at dinner."

"Sounds good to me."

They take the elevator up to the restaurant and get a table next to the window where they can see the outline of the city. Aceline is now wearing a low-cut black evening gown and David again marvels at the transformation in her appearance. "When I first saw you come through the lobby, I had to take a second look to make sure it was you. All I can say is that you clean up nicely."

"I guess I'll take that as a compliment."

"I meant to say you look fantastic."

"Thank you. It is amazing what nice clothes and a little makeup can do."

"I didn't realize this was a luxury hotel. I guess I need to go out tomorrow and get some better threads."

"You look fine, but I would be happy to go shopping with you tomorrow if you like."

"I look forward to it. Have you been to Casablanca before?"

"When I was married. My ex and I came here twice, mainly because he liked to gamble. While I have no interest in gambling, I found the country to be very interesting. There is an energy in the city that you can feel day and night. The architecture is magical — it has intricate designs in the tiles you see throughout the city. They are everywhere, including the walls, floors and water pools. The open markets are fun to explore and the food is excellent and unique, particularly since groups of people tend to gather and eat from one super-sized communal plate. I'm excited to show you some of what makes Morocco special."

The waiter comes over and asks if they are ready to order drinks and dinner. Aceline asks David if she should order for the both of them and he nods "yes". She orders *harira*, a Moroccan tomato-based soup laden with rice. For the entree, she selects lamb with various vegetables and steamed couscous grains, along with mint tea. She isn't sure if David will like the tea since it is very sweet. She decides to order it anyway as tea is a national obsession, and many Moroccan citizens drink it multiple times each day. The waiter smiles and tells Aceline she has made excellent choices.

Aceline turns her attention back to David. "Tell me about your trip to Brazil."

"It was both concerning and thought-provoking. The Zika virus outbreak is mainly limited to a few provinces in Brazil at this point, but seems to be spreading rapidly to other provinces and countries. The incidence of congenital abnormalities in pregnant women infected with the virus is still not clear but is likely around 10%. Efforts are ongoing to develop drugs to treat the virus, but since it usually does not cause symptoms, it is very hard to see how drugs will be the answer. The work on vaccines has been going on for less than a year. To date, the most promising vaccine is a vector vaccine that uses a live, but weakened dengue virus, to produce a Zika virus protein that could protect against infection. There is a lot of discussion about whether this type of vaccine could ever be used in pregnant women."

"Why is that? We are using the live virus yellow fever vaccine in the current yellow fever outbreak in the DRC and almost all the pregnant women decided they want it."

"There are several major differences between the two vaccines. The mortality rate in pregnant women with yellow fever is substantial, while there is no mortality in women infected with the Zika virus. Additionally, we have a considerable amount of safety data with the yellow fever vaccine in pregnant women who inadvertently received the vaccine, and there were no reported problems in them or their unborn child. The only experience we have with a vector vaccine was with the Ebola vaccine used towards the end of the Ebola outbreak in Western Africa. In this Ebola outbreak, we tried to exclude pregnant women from getting the vaccine, although about two dozen women were inadvertently given the vaccine and did not reveal any serious side effects."

"I get the differences between using the yellow fever vaccine and a vector vaccine, but I think many women would want to use the vaccine if it would protect their baby from being infected with the Zika virus. It seems to me they could inform pregnant women of potential risks to themselves or their baby, but let them make the decision for themselves."

"Funny you should say that. Venetia Sousa is one of the researchers I met in Brazil. She is involved with planning a Phase 2 study with the vaccine and that is exactly how she feels. In fact, she is currently pregnant and worried about whether the Zika virus will affect her baby. She told me that she plans to get the vaccine as part of the Phase 2 study."

"Has she been tested yet to see if she has been infected by the virus?"

"Yes, but the results were inconclusive and she wants to do all she can to protect her baby if she is not already infected."

The waiter brings the mint tea and soup to their table. Aceline updates David on the expanded yellow fever vaccination campaign and that the number of cases seems to be decreasing. The dinner lasts over two hours and Aceline tells David she thinks they both need to get some sleep. David wonders if she plans to go to his room, but as they get on the elevator, the answer becomes clear as Aceline pushes the button for her floor and asks what time they should meet for breakfast. David is disappointed but hopes her decision is due to her long day of travel. When David gets to his room, he lies down on the bed and turns on the television, as he does most nights.

***

The next morning, he wakes up in the clothes he wore to dinner. He looks at his watch and notices he has only 30 minutes before he needs to meet Aceline for breakfast. He showers quickly, throws on some clothes, and rushes down to the hotel lobby where Aceline is waiting.

"David, what do you think about getting breakfast as we walk around Casablanca?"

"Sounds good to me. How did you sleep?"

"Like a baby. I'm rested and ready to explore the city with you. Do you want to walk to the Hassan II Mosque? It's a little over a mile away and I was thinking we could get breakfast along the way?"

They start walking and Aceline wraps her arm around his elbow. David wonders if this makes her feel more secure or is actually a romantic gesture. He smiles at her and keeps his arm in place as they continue walking down the street. Halfway to the Hassan II Mosque, they sit down for breakfast at an outdoor café.

"Can you give me an overview of the history of Casablanca?"

Aceline pauses for a moment. "Have you ever seen the movie Casablanca starring Humphrey Bogart?"

"I have and liked it so much that I have seen it several times over the years."

"Same here. After seeing the movie, I read a book on the history of Casablanca. I am far from an expert on this topic, but given you previously told me you are a history buff, I reviewed the history on Wikipedia on the flight here."

"Wow! You read my mind."

"The history of Casablanca traces back to the 10th century. Back then the town's name was Anfa, now one of the city's suburbs. For several centuries before and after this time, various Arab Islamic sects waged holy wars against one another. In the 13th century, Anfa came under the influence of the Marinid dynasty, but eventually became independent as the dynasty weakened."

"Really? Based on the movie Casablanca, I thought the country was under European rule for many centuries. Am I off base?"

"Actually, Portugal, then France ruled Casablanca, but that came after the Marinid dynasty. The Portuguese destroyed the town in the mid-15th century as reprisal for ongoing piracy. They sent a fleet of vessels and a large contingent of soldiers to occupy the town. They ransacked the town but later abandoned it. Piracy again flared up in the early 16th century, and the Portuguese returned and once again destroyed the rebuilt town. The Portuguese rebuilt the town in the later part of the 16th century and renamed it Casa Branca in an attempt to establish control over the area. Muslim tribes attacked the Portuguese rulers frequently and eventually, Portugal abandoned the town following a major earthquake in the middle of the 18th century."

"For some reason, I thought France was here during that time. When did France get involved?"

"In the early 20th century. The French attempted to build a railway near the city's port, but the local population attacked them. Riots ensued, and the French bombarded the city from ships off the coast and then landed troops inside the town. This attack resulted in over 15,000 casualties and severe damage to the town. The French claimed the city to restore order and this began the process of colonization. The French conquest of Morocco took place in 1911 with the Treaty of Fez, formally turning control of Morocco over to France."

"Wow! Quite the tumultuous history. I know Morocco is no longer under French rule. How did that happen?"

"The movie highlights the city's colonial status at the time, depicting it as the scene of a power struggle between competing European powers. Europeans formed almost half the population. During the 1940s and 1950s, Casablanca was a major center of anti-French riots. A bomb attack on Christmas Day in 1953 resulted in 16 deaths. This uprising led to the French-Moroccan Agreement, which gave Morocco independence from France in 1956."

"What does that mean for Casablanca now?"

"Currently, Casablanca has a population of over three million people and is the main center for business and commerce in Morocco. The city has modern facilities, good roads, a railway system leading to other parts of the country, as well as the largest artificial ports in the world. Over 95% of the population is Sunnis. Berber — a Moroccan dialect of Arabic — and French are the most common languages spoken."

Aceline's depth of knowledge impresses David. "Wow! I could read ten books on the history of Casablanca and not remember anywhere near what you just told me. I'll pay for breakfast and we can head to the mosque."

David and Aceline walk along the shoreline through the northern end of the older part of the city. The maze of alleyways proves to be a great place to experience the pulse of Casablanca life, including tradesmen selling various wares to shoppers. When they arrive at the mosque at the edge of the bay, its beauty startles David.

Aceline continues to share her in-depth knowledge of the city. "The mosque was completed in 1993. It is the second-largest mosque in the world and has the world's tallest minaret, which is 200 meters high."

"What is a minaret?"

"The minaret is a tall, slender tower that is part of every mosque. Projecting galleries surround the minaret and this is where the muezzin, the person who chants the call for prayer, announces the prayer to worshippers.

"The architecture of the mosque has intricate mixtures of tiles, marble, and stone, with multiple colors including blue, white and gold. The prayer hall can accommodate around 25,000 worshippers and the courtyard has a retractable roof and can hold another 80,000 people."

"That's incredible."

They walk around the mosque for over an hour before going to a nearby restaurant for lunch. They choose an outdoor table and David is really craving a cold beer. "It would be great if you would order for both of us, but I would like a beer if possible."

"Morocco, unlike some other Muslim countries, does allow liquor to be served in restaurants, but not around religious sites."

"Damn, I guess it will be mint tea then."

Aceline orders their lunch and then wants to change the conversation to learn more about David. "You know I was thinking about you the other day and I realized you rarely talk about your childhood or what made you decide to have a career in global health."

David flushes slightly and then begins to tell his story. "You were thinking about me, huh? Well, I was born in a rural town in northern Australia where my parents who were physicians worked to improve the health of the indigenous aboriginal population. I was their only child and was very close to my parents. Early on, I decided I wanted to become a physician. I wanted to make the world a better place by improving the health of disadvantaged people and felt that my education was key to doing this. Upon graduating from the University of Queensland School of Medicine, I did an internal medicine residency and infectious disease fellowship at Queensland Medical Center. After that, I decided I wasn't quite done with school and decided to attend the London School of Hygiene and Tropical Medicine where I obtained a Master's degree in Public Health and Policy. I then joined the WHO and spent the last 12 years working in countries experiencing various types of infectious disease outbreaks, including yellow fever in Africa and South America, cholera in Africa, Asia and the Americas, and most recently, Ebola in Western Africa where we met."

"Your parents sound like they were wonderful people. I'd love to hear more about them."

Aceline is very surprised as his eyes become moist. "I rarely talk about my parents because their death is very painful memory. In 2010, I was working in the cholera outbreak in Haiti. One day, I got a call from a close friend of mine working at the WHO. He told me my parents were involved in a car accident and both of them had died. I rushed home to Australia in time for the funeral, but since then have felt an emptiness within me. My work has helped fill this void, since I believe they would be proud of the work I am doing. I am not sure if this makes any sense, but I think that part of the reason I agreed to take the Interim-Director of the Human Emergencies Program position, is to continue to honor the work they did to help those most in need."

Aceline reaches out and holds David's hand. She had previously heard that his parents had died in an accident, but until this moment had not realized this had occurred during the past decade, nor the impact it had on David. She feels terrible she gave him a hard time when he told her he was accepting the position. "I'm so sorry that you had to go through this tragedy. I am glad that you shared this with me. Let's finish eating and then go someplace that reminds us of the restorative aspects of life."

David and Aceline go to Place Mohamed V in the central plaza of Casablanca. The area has a fountain and beautiful gardens. After spending a few hours there, Aceline can tell that David's mood has lightened up.

"David, there are some nice clothing shops for men in this part of town. Are you up for going shopping?"

"Sure. Will you help me pick out the clothes that I can wear here?"

"You have a deal."

They walk to a nearby open-air market and at one of the stalls Aceline suggests some clothes David might like. He buys two cotton-collared shirts and a pair of white linen pants she picks out.

"Do you like these clothes or are you buying them just because I like them?" Aceline asks.

He puts his arm over her shoulder. "I never went shopping for clothes before with a woman other than my mom and I'm enjoying the experience. I might not have picked them out if I was shopping alone, but I like them and want you to like what I wear."

"That's an honest answer. Are you willing to reciprocate and help me pick out some clothes?"

"I am, but you are under no obligation to choose what I pick out."

They continue shopping at several other booths and Aceline buys a cotton dress that David likes and a pair of sandals. As the evening approaches, David notes the area is becoming more crowded with families walking on the streets. "Do families often come here at night?"

"Some are here for dinner or other reasons, but many families just enjoy strolling through the area."

"Would you like to eat dinner at one of the nearby restaurants?"

"That would be great. There are a lot of restaurants close by in Ain Diab, which is the main beach in Casablanca. If we go now, we should be able to find a restaurant that offers us a view of the Atlantic Ocean while we dine."

They decide to eat at Boccaccio, a restaurant that specializes in Italian food. The menu looks good, but David wonders if they should get wine with their meal.

"Can we order wine here and, if so, what would you suggest?"

"Morocco is a leading wine-producing country and some of the vineyards are on the Casablanca coast. My favorite local red wine is Bonaassia, which has a blackcurrant taste."

Along with the Bonaassia, David orders manicotti and Aceline gets a lasagna. While eating, Aceline decides to see if David is willing to discuss their relationship.

"David, before you left the DRC to travel to Brazil, you told me you wanted to move our relationship beyond friendship. Are you willing to share your thoughts with me on how you hope our relationship might evolve?"

David mulls over her question. "That's a loaded question, but I will admit I have given it a fair amount of thought, especially while I was in Brazil. I think it would be helpful if I describe the relationship between my parents in their professional and personal lives. The way they interacted with each other professionally was very different than at home. They were very serious when working and you would never guess that they were married. However, they were warm and playful at home, not only with me, but with each other and you could see how much they loved each other. Their ability to separate work and home is something I want and need."

"Their relationship sounds amazing. The more you tell me about your parents, the more I wish I could have known them. Have you ever had a relationship with a woman where you came close to that?"

"I had only two long-term relationships with women and neither of them came close to that. I have often wondered if what was missing in those previous relationships was my fault, but all I can tell you is that they felt I did not pay enough attention to them. That is likely a fair assessment, but I am also certain I did not love them."

"What, if anything, makes you think our relationship can reach that point?"

"From a work standpoint, we are already there, at least in my mind. I have tremendous respect for what you achieve at work and I like the fact that you have no problems letting me know when I do something you think is wrong. My parents did that at work and yet never brought any of those issues home."

Aceline likes his response but wants to know about the non-work part of their relationship. "What do you hope for in our personal life?"

"I want it to be one where we are best friends who are also lovers. The bond would be so strong that both of us would prefer being home."

"Can you give me more insight into what you mean?"

"A good example would be: When we are away from each other traveling for work, we can't wait to come home."

"Do you think this is truly possible?"

"I know it's possible. I grew up in that household. Can I ask you some questions about what went wrong in your marriage and what you hope for in our relationship?"

"Fair enough. Daniel and I got married in 2004 after dating for less than six months. Initially, the marriage seemed good, but I soon found out he started seeing other women soon after we were married. When I confronted him about this, he told me that men aren't meant to be monogamous. I threw him out of our apartment that night and haven't had anything to do with him since."

"Has time helped ease the pain or are you still dealing with the hurt?"

"That's a fair question. I am definitely over Daniel, but it has left me with some doubts about my ability to judge a man's character. In retrospect, there were things I should have noticed during the six-month courtship.

"Such as?"

"Some of the things he would say pointed to his belief that the man needed to control the relationship."

"What do you need from me in a relationship?"

"A lot of what I want is similar to what you just described — love, a deep friendship, respect, equality, and perhaps most of all, honesty."

Their dinner conversation continues to focus on what each other needs in a relationship. The time flies by. Eventually, they take a taxi back to the hotel and as they enter the hotel lobby, David wonders what to do next. "Would you like to get a drink at the bar?"

"David, today has been a really enjoyable and remarkable day. However, I really need to get some sleep. Would you like to spend some time at the beach and visit the vineyards tomorrow?"

"That sounds like fun."

"Great, let's meet in the lobby at 9 a.m."

David goes to his room. He changes into his pajamas and lies in bed. He thinks the discussion about their relationship was interesting, but he is still unsure if Aceline is interested in pursuing a romantic relationship with him. Different thoughts keep circulating in his brain, but he soon falls into a deep sleep.

***

The following morning David goes to the hotel lobby where Aceline is waiting for him with a big smile. "I am glad to see you smiling this morning. You must have slept well last night."

"It took me a while to fall asleep because I was thinking about all of our conversations yesterday, but once I fell asleep, I was out cold. As I woke up this morning, I realized I had a dream about you."

"I hope it was a good dream."

"It was. Maybe I will tell you more about it tonight?"

"I look forward to hearing the details."

Aceline suggests they have breakfast at the hotel and then spend the rest of the morning at the beach and the afternoon visiting a few wine vineyards along the coast. The conversation throughout the day is casual. David wonders where they should go for dinner.

"Today was really fun. Would you like to go out for dinner or eat in the hotel?"

"Actually, I was thinking about us going back to the hotel and getting room service."

"I like that idea. Shall we dine in your room or mine?"

"We should be back at the hotel by 5 p.m. Why don't you come to my room at 7 p.m. and I can order room service."

When David gets back to his room, he glimpses at the 57 emails sent to him that day. He decides none of them requires his immediate attention. He wants to take a nap and sets his alarm so that he has time to shower before he heads down to Aceline's room. Lying in bed, he ponders the various parts of Aceline's personality that he likes but never took time to appreciate. He knew she was very smart, but her diverse interests and extensive knowledge about non-medical topics are new to him. That, combined with her zest and optimism about life, makes him appreciate her even more. The next thing he knows his alarm is ringing and he gets up to shower, and puts on a blue shirt and white pants he purchased yesterday.

He goes to her room and knocks on the door. Aceline opens the door in black lingerie. Before he can utter more than the word "WOW", she pulls him into the room and wraps her arms around him. He holds her tightly as they passionately kiss. He pulls the straps off her shoulders and the lingerie falls to the floor, while she unbuttons his shirt and pants. He picks her up and carries her to the bed and she moans gently as his hands roam over her body. When he is inside her, they seem to be moving as one and eventually they climax together. After they lie facing each other, he feels content and hopes she feels the same.

David looks into her eyes, "I thought about this moment many times, but was never sure it would happen."

"This was my dream last night and I'm really glad it did. We can talk more about us later, but right now I'm starving and we need to order room service before it gets too late."

**

When they get out of bed the following day, it is almost noon. The weather outside is sunny and warmer than usual for this time of the year. Aceline suggests they hire a car and spend the day in El Jadida, a town on the southern Atlantic coast about an hour away from Casablanca. When they arrive in El Jadida, they go to the Citadel area built by the Portuguese. They explore an old prison and then stop at a café for lunch. In the afternoon, they visit the cisterns.

"The cisterns were built in the 16th century as an armory but were later made into a water reservoir," Aceline notes. "Very little outside light gets into the cisterns and they are dark and wet due to an overflowing pool in the center."

They next walk along the seawall holding hands and enjoy the spectacular sea views.

"David, what do you think of the area?"

"This town is really interesting, but the cisterns are kind of creepy."

"They remind me of the catacombs in Paris I visited when I was a child," Aceline remarks.

"You're right. Both the cisterns and catacombs give me the feeling of being in a horror film."

"Are you okay?"

"I'm with you and that makes everything okay."

"That's really sweet. I admire a lot of things about you, but I would have never guessed that you had a romantic side."

"To be honest, neither did I, but you bring out a whole load of feelings that are new to me."

"What do you say to heading back to the hotel and see what other emotions I can find?"

"That would be the perfect end to an already wonderful day."

***

David and Aceline spend the rest of the week exploring other sites in Morocco as well as each other. On the last night, David decides he needs to see if he can bring some clarity to how to keep this relationship moving forward.

"I can't believe how fast the week has gone by. I have to go to Geneva tomorrow to update the Director-General about the Zika virus outbreak in Brazil. Can you come with me?"

"I need to return to the DRC so that one of the other nurses can go on vacation. I do have additional vacation time — perhaps we can spend the winter holidays together?"

"Fantastic. Do you want to meet in Geneva or somewhere else?"

"Let me think about it."

"I'm going to miss you big time."

"Same here, but let's not waste the rest of the night talking."

Chapter 6

Geneva, Switzerland
Late October 2016

The next day, David travels to Geneva and upon landing at the airport, he turns on his cell phone. A number of text messages appear and he notices one is from the Director-General's office asking him to meet with her and others in the WHO leadership group today at 5 p.m. He responds that he may be a little late, but will be there as soon as possible. He gets through the immigration line in less than 20 minutes, picks up his luggage, and hails a taxi for the short trip to the WHO headquarters.

David reaches the conference room at 5:10 p.m. and knocks on the door. The Director-General thanks him for coming at short notice and requests he gives the group an overview of what he has learned while in Brazil. He highlights his major findings, noting that the Zika virus outbreak is occurring in multiple provinces in Brazil and is spreading into some of the other countries in South America, Latin America, the Caribbean, and most recently the southern end of Florida in the United States (US). The best estimate suggests approximately 10% of pregnant women infected with the virus are giving birth to infants with microcephaly and/or other abnormalities. Usually, these findings are noticeable at birth, but in some cases don't appear until later in infancy. The CDC and other organizations have redirected funding to support epidemiologic studies as well as the development of drugs and vaccines. He highlights that the first Phase 2 vaccine study in healthy adults is in the planning stage in Brazil and will use a vector vaccine, but this study does not include any pregnant women. He promises to share his full report with everyone as soon as it is finished. He then opens the floor for questions.

The Director-General thanks David for the overview and then asks the first question, "What are the most important things the WHO can do to help?"

"There are currently no vaccines or drugs available for the prevention or treatment of the Zika virus. This is not surprising given that for other diseases, very few drugs and no vaccines have been studied in pregnant women prior to being approved by the US Food and Drug Administration, European Medicines Agency, or other regulatory agencies. For infectious disease outbreaks, this problem has become more severe as the number of outbreaks has increased. Recent epidemics, including those due to yellow fever, Zika, Ebola, and H1N1 influenza viruses provide ample proof that these viruses can severely affect the health of pregnant women and their offspring. Indeed, for each of these viruses, pregnant women are at a significantly higher risk of serious disease and death than non-pregnant women of similar age. Infection in pregnancy can also result in death or severe abnormalities in the fetus. The ongoing yellow fever outbreak in the DRC has brought this problem to a head, and SAGE recently felt compelled to recommend the off-label use of the live virus yellow fever vaccine to pregnant women in the DRC."

The Director-General asks a follow-up question. "Your points are well taken. However, in the current Zika virus outbreak, we are dealing with a disease whose major consequence is not to the pregnant woman, but her unborn child. Does this affect your willingness to use the vaccine in pregnant women?"

"Not really. I believe that many pregnant women would volunteer to participate in this type of vaccine study since it has the potential to protect their unborn child."

Dr. Sara Alverez, the Director of the Maternal and Child Health Division, asks the next question. "Why not give the Zika vaccine to young adolescent females prior to the time they become sexually active. We do this for the human papilloma virus (HPV) vaccine to prevent cervical cancer that will occur decades later."

"I see several issues with this approach. First, if we only give the vaccine to young adolescent females, this will not protect women who are currently of an age where they can become pregnant. Second, we now know that the HPV vaccine provides protection for more than a decade, and perhaps for a lifetime. In contrast, we have no idea of the duration of the protection of the Zika virus vaccine. Unless the Zika virus vaccine provides protection for decades, the vaccine will still need to be given to women at an age where they might become pregnant. Finally, I believe there is a compelling ethical argument that pregnant women have the right to decide whether they want to participate in studies examining vaccines and drugs that are potentially beneficial to themselves and their baby."

Dr. Alverez more adamantly expresses her concerns, "I understand your points, but remain very concerned about using a new vaccine in pregnant women until there is substantial experience with its use in the general population. I would be interested in hearing your arguments in favor of doing this."

"We must find a way to overcome the reluctance of pharmaceutical companies, governments and others to do the necessary studies in and for pregnant women. The companies don't do the studies needed to determine whether the drugs are safe and efficacious in pregnant women because they are worried about their legal risks if the baby has a problem at birth, whether or not the problem was due to the vaccine or drug. Therefore, regulatory agencies have not labeled the majority of drugs and vaccines for use by pregnant women. However, these drugs and vaccines are frequently used off-label by physicians to prevent or treat various health problems in pregnant women. We must find a way to overcome the reluctance to do the necessary studies for pregnant women. If we can't break through this barrier, we will never have the same quality, safety and efficacy data we have for other groups that get the vaccine."

Dr. Cynthia Edwards, a pediatrician, discusses a similar issue that occurred in children. "Until the turn of this current century, children faced a similar problem where most drugs used to treat their illnesses were being used off-label."

Someone interjects, "I've heard 'off-label' multiple times, but I'm not sure what that means."

Dr. Edwards continues, "By off-label, I mean the companies making these drugs had studied them for optimal dose, safety and efficacy in adults, but not in children. Therefore, the regulatory agencies would label these drugs for use in adults, but not for children. This puts pediatricians and other healthcare professionals caring for children in the very difficult position of having to use these drugs without the needed information. Starting in the 1980s, the American Academy of Pediatrics lobbied the US Congress to fix this issue. In 2003, Congress passed the Best Pharmaceuticals for Children Act and Pediatric Research Equity Act. Pharmaceutical companies are now doing these studies, resulting in many of the drugs now being used on-label in children in the US and many other countries. Similar to children, I believe pregnant women deserve drugs and vaccines that are known to be safe and effective in them."

David then adds, "Cynthia, I agree with everything you said. I spent the last decade dealing with various outbreaks, and aside from the 2009 influenza pandemic, pregnant women were denied the opportunity to receive vaccines that could protect them and their offspring from the ravages of these diseases. The Zika virus is somewhat different in that the fetus is the only one at risk of a severe outcome from the virus. However, many countries have recently started to immunize pregnant women with acellular pertussis vaccines to help protect young infants against whooping cough. I feel certain many mothers would want the chance to protect their baby against the Zika virus if a safe and effective vaccine was available."

The Director-General asks, "David, what do you think the WHO can do to move this issue forward?"

"We must proactively consider the interests of pregnant women and their babies in research and development efforts to combat epidemic threats. This is especially true for vaccines, an essential tool for decreasing the impact of infectious disease outbreaks. I think we need to convene a group of experts in the areas of bioethics, infectious diseases, obstetrics, pediatrics, and regulatory approval processes to consider the various issues and make recommendations."

The Director-General realizes the conversation has been heated and intense and decides to end the meeting. She asks David to come back to her office to continue this discussion regarding pregnant women. "David, I want to thank you for coming to the meeting on such short notice. How was your vacation?"

"I spent a wonderful week in Morocco."

"That's terrific. It makes me feel better, since after we finish this discussion I need to ask you to go on another trip. I think you made a compelling case for the need to do these studies in pregnant women. I agree that the first step is for the WHO to put together a group of outside experts to provide guidance on how best to do this. Do you think one advisory group can do this for both vaccines and drugs?"

"My guess is that several advisory groups will be needed since the ethical and regulatory considerations for vaccines versus drugs are substantially different. The advisory groups will also have to think about how to incorporate pregnant women into ongoing studies for new vaccines that are under development."

"Which new vaccines are you talking about?"

"In addition to Zika virus, these include eight other viral diseases the WHO listed late last year as our top priority for research and development.

"Remind me which eight are on the list."

"Crimean Congo hemorrhagic fever, Ebola, Marburg disease, Lassa fever, Nipah and Rift Valley fever, as well as the two coronaviruses that cause severe acute respiratory disease (SARS-1) and the Middle East respiratory syndrome (MERS). While there are research groups and companies working to develop vaccines and treatments for these diseases, based on previous experience, it is highly unlikely studies will include pregnant women."

"Got it. I will add this issue to the next meeting of the WHO Secretariat Leadership Council and seek their advice. Based on the discussion after your presentation today, it seems not everyone will be in favor of doing studies on pregnant women. However, I think what happened in the 2014 Ebola outbreak in West Africa and the current outbreak of the Zika virus makes a powerful argument for forming these advisory groups. They can provide recommendations on a range of pregnancy-specific issues, including under what circumstances pregnant women should receive vaccines for these types of diseases and what specific information pregnant women need prior to offering them a vaccine."

"Thank you. I think the advisory groups can also provide advice on what the WHO can do to encourage pharmaceutical companies to perform the needed studies in pregnant women."

"I will work with the leadership team to decide how best to implement this process and will keep you up to date on what we decide. In the meantime, I need you to travel to Atlanta and meet with Dr. Richard Huff, the new Interim-Director of the CDC, to learn about the work they are doing in conjunction with the Chinese CDC on the emergence of an H7N9 bird strain of influenza virus that is causing disease in humans in Asia. While you are there, you can get an update on their plans for dealing with the Zika virus outbreak in the US."

"I didn't realize the previous CDC Director is no longer there."

"He resigned after Donald Trump was elected President of the US."

"What do you know about the new Director?"

"He worked in the CDC Influenza Division and oversaw the US planning process for the 2009 influenza pandemic. Since then, he's worked on the US planning process for the next flu pandemic and has also been collaborating with us on the Influenza Pandemic Global Action Plan."

"Anything else you need me to find out?"

"I am hearing from some of our financial supporters that the US President-elect is considering cutting back financial support for global health. Any information you can get about cutbacks, including those that might occur to the CDC's Global Health Division budget, would be helpful."

"Oh boy. All right, I will make sure to ask. I will have my office make the necessary travel arrangements and get back to you once I know more."

"Thank you and have a safe trip."

Chapter 7

Centers for Disease Control and Prevention Atlanta, US, November 2016, Day 1

D avid arrives at the Atlanta airport two days later and takes a taxi to the CDC headquarters. It has been many years since he last visited the CDC and he is amazed at how much the campus has changed. There are many new buildings and the security to enter the CDC has markedly increased. Although Richard Huff's assistant, Melinda, meets him at the main entrance to the CDC, he is still required to go through a screening process similar to those at airports. He finally receives a badge after 20 minutes, and Melinda escorts him to the office where Richard is waiting for him.

"David, it is nice to meet you. I heard from colleagues in the CDC Global Division that your work on various global outbreaks has been stellar."

"Thanks. I've heard great things about you too and I'm hoping to learn a lot from you and others at the CDC. I can't believe how much the CDC campus has grown since I was last here in the early 2000s."

"Probably a good way to start would be for us to go to Building 21 that houses the CDC Emergency Outbreak Center — it was built after you were last here."

They pass through several other security checkpoints before arriving at a very large room that contains the Emergency Operating Center. David notices a theater size screen in the front with a map of the globe and multiple lights flashing. Over two dozen people are sitting in front of their computers.

Richard starts to explain the origin and functions of the Emergency Operating Center. "The first time someone enters this area they often remark how it reminds them of the US space center they see on television during launches of space crafts. The need for a dedicated Emergency Outbreak Center in the CDC became clear early this century after someone sent the bacteria that causes anthrax through the mail to various people and the World Trade Center terrorist attack. Soon thereafter, the Emergency Outbreak Center facility plan was developed, and the center became operational early in 2006.

"This building is different than others that I have seen."

"You're right. They did not spare a cent on this building, as the Emergency Outbreak Center is a 24,000-square-foot facility that can seat as many as 230 people at a time. The CDC employees who work in the Emergency Operating Center receive extensive training that prepares them to detect, monitor and respond to possible new public health events. These same individuals are on call to support a response should one be needed. The head of the Emergency Operating Center is not here right now, but he is on your visit agenda to meet this afternoon."

"Does the Emergency Operating Center function throughout the year?"

"Even when there is no ongoing public health threat, the Emergency Outbreak Center has dedicated staff monitoring information, 24 hours a day, 365 days a year. The Center monitors potential public health threats through its watch desk, which takes calls from physicians, state and local authorities, and the public. Notifications also come via public health partner briefings, field operations intelligence, or a WHO declaration of a Public Health Emergency of International Concern. If the threat appears significant, a team with expertise on the particular subject determines whether to activate the Incident Management System. The team's assessment goes to the CDC director and other leadership in the government who provide recommendations for action."

"During a public health emergency, the Emergency Outbreak Center deploys scientific experts, coordinates the delivery of supplies and equipment to the incident site, monitors response activities, and provides resources to state and local public health departments. The Incident Management System has been activated continuously since December 2011."

"What events are currently being monitored in the Emergency Operating Center?"

"We continuously monitor influenza outbreaks including the avian H5N1 outbreak first detected in Hong Kong in 1997 and the H7N9 outbreak that began in China in 2013. Currently, we are also monitoring the Zika virus outbreak in various countries in the Americas and lead contamination of drinking water in Flint, Michigan."

"The first two of those are exactly what the WHO Director-General wants me to explore with you on this visit. I don't know anything about the lead drinking water problem, but perhaps you can tell me about it later."

Richard waves at someone in the back of the room and then walks with David to where she is standing. "David, let me introduce you to Elena Sanchez who is leading the Emergency Outbreak Center group monitoring the Zika virus outbreak. She will be meeting with you tomorrow to update you on the epidemiology of the Zika virus outbreak in the Americas and what plans they are considering to intervene."

David shakes Elena's hand while telling her he has many questions for her and looks forward to talking with her.

Richard then takes David over to the area on the campus containing the Biohazard buildings. David is struck by the size of the building. Richard tells David that the 400,000-square-foot, concrete facility is one of only about a dozen such facilities within the US with a Biosafety level-4 (BSL-4) laboratory. "David, are you interested in knowing about what is done in the BSL-4 levels we have in this facility?"

"Yes, if it isn't too much of a hassle?"

"No problem. I will ask Eric Moser who supervises this facility to tell us about it." Richard sends a quick text on his phone and Eric comes up from the floor below them. Richard introduces him to David. Eric then begins to explain what determines the level of biosafety required in a particular laboratory.

"Biosafety levels (BSL) 1–4 designate what precautions are required to works with various types of microbes. At the lowest level is biosafety (BSL-1), the laboratories are studying microbes, such as *Lactobacillus acidophilus*, which have a low risk for causing serious problems for personnel or the environment, and precautions consist of regular hand-washing and minimal protective equipment. At the highest level (BSL-4), the microbes being studied are of very high risk to personnel or others if they are released into the environment. The BSL-4 laboratories are specially designed to ensure the safety of those working there. There are also established protocols for all procedures, extensive personnel training, and high levels of security to control access to the facility. The security and safety features are similar to what one might see in science fiction movies. There are biometric security devices, including iris scans and fingerprinting for those entering the high-containment laboratories."

Before Eric goes any further, David asks, "Can you give me some examples of what microbes would be studied in the various BSL-4 laboratories?"

"BSL-4 laboratories are required for diagnostic work and research on easily transmitted pathogens that can cause fatal diseases, such as the Ebola virus and the anthrax bacteria that was used in a domestic terrorist attack just one week after the Al-Qaeda terrorist plane attack on September 11, 2001."

"It has been a long time since I thought about the anthrax attack. Can you remind me of what happened?"

"Bruce Edwards Ivins, a scientist at the government's biodefense laboratories at Fort Detrick in Maryland, is believed to be the person who initiated the anthrax terrorist attack. Over a period of several weeks, he sent a fine white powder containing anthrax spores to several news outlets and various politicians. Seventeen people inhaled the spores through the respiratory route, resulting in them developing pneumonia. They received antibiotics, but five people died."

"What happened to Bruce Ivins?"

"The Federal Bureau of Investigation (FBI) investigated the case over the next seven years. Initially, Steve Hatfill, a bioweapons expert, was the primary suspect, but eventually was exonerated. Ivins became the primary suspect around 2005, but committed suicide before he was formally charged."

"Thanks — I remember hearing about that now, but never heard how it ended. Are you still studying anthrax in this facility?"

"Currently, we are focused on the Ebola virus, which caused over 11,000 deaths in Western Africa a few years ago and also infected a small number of Americans."

"How many US citizens were diagnosed with an Ebola virus infection?"

"There were seven US citizens working in Africa who were diagnosed with an Ebola infection and evacuated to the US. Two other US citizens were diagnosed with Ebola in this country, but they contracted the disease overseas. Additionally, two nurses caring for Ebola patients in the US developed an Ebola infection. Two of the patients who contracted the disease overseas died while being cared for in the US.

"Would it be possible for me to go inside the BSL-4 laboratory?"

"I would be happy to show you the BSL-4 laboratory in Building 17 through a window in a room that separates the laboratory from non-restricted areas. It will take us about 30 to 45 minutes though. Do you have the time?"

David looks at Richard and he indicates that it is fine. Richard asks Eric to bring David to his office once they are finished.

Eric takes David to the room where he can look through the window into the BSL-4 laboratory. Eric explains some of the features.

"BSL-4 laboratories must be separated from areas with unrestricted traffic. The airflow design ensures air always flows from clean areas of the laboratory to areas where the microbes are studied. The entrance to the BSL-4 laboratory uses airlocks to help prevent aerosols from escaping from the laboratory. All laboratory waste, including filtered air, water and trash must also be decontaminated before it can leave the facility.

"Wow, this really does look like a scene from a sci-fi movie. The staff working inside look like they are wearing space suits."

"Indeed, they are wearing positive-pressure equipment similar to what astronauts wear when leaving a rocket or space station. The cabinets where the staff members are working have seamless edges to make cleaning easier and reduce the chance of someone tearing their gloves. The airflow in the cabinets takes the microbes through a system that filters and kills all germs before leaving the building. Decontamination of materials used by the staff occurs before leaving the cabinet area by passing through a tank of disinfectant."

"What happens when they need to take a break or leave for the day?"

"Anytime they leave the BSL-4 laboratory, the staff must pass through a chemical shower for decontamination, then a room for removing the positive-pressure suit, followed by a personal shower. Entry into the BSL-4 laboratory is restricted to trained and authorized individuals, and all persons entering and exiting the laboratory are recorded.

"Thanks, Eric, this was incredibly informative."

"Glad to do it. I can answer any other questions you have while we walk back to Dr. Huff's office."

David arrives outside Richard's office ten minutes later. Richard waves for him to come inside. "Would you like something to drink or eat?"

"Tea would be great. The tour was amazing. I still can't believe how much the CDC campus has grown since I was last here. The Emergency Outbreak Center is impressive; I may incorporate some of the Center's methods into our surveillance systems in Geneva. How much time do we have together today?"

"Here is a copy of the schedule for your two-day visit. We created it based on what your administrative assistant told us. I set aside the rest of the afternoon for us to talk and scheduled a dinner meeting for us tomorrow night. You also have multiple meetings with CDC people who are knowledgeable in the areas you are interested in learning more about. If you need any changes made to the agenda, just let me know."

David reviews the agenda. "The agenda looks good. The Director-General asked me to find out more about what the CDC is doing to deal with the emergence of the Zika virus in the Americas and the status of the avian flu virus outbreaks in China. I appreciate you allowing me to spend considerable time with the CDC Zika virus group and some of the members of the Global Division. My understanding is that you were the Head of the CDC Influenza Division prior to this? If you are still connected to that work, it would be great if you would update me on the recent avian influenza outbreak in Asia."

"How much experience do you have with avian influenza outbreaks?"

"Most of my career has been spent dealing with other types of outbreaks, including Ebola, yellow fever, and cholera. My knowledge about avian influenza is definitely not at the same level. However, I spent most of my time on the plane trip from Geneva to Atlanta refreshing my understanding of the various types of influenza viruses and their role in human and animal disease. Would it be okay if I ask you a list of questions I have and then you can fill in any other information that you think I am missing?"

"Sounds good."

"My understanding is that there are two types of influenza viruses, A and B, which cause significant human disease. These viruses have two proteins on the outside of the virus membrane. The hemagglutinin (H) protein helps the virus attach to cells in the respiratory tract where the virus can replicate. The neuraminidase (N) protein enables the newly formed viruses to detach from the cell and continue to spread and infect additional respiratory tract cells. It seems like there are many different types of hemagglutinins and neuraminidases, but not all of them are found in humans. Is that correct?"

"Yes. For influenza A viruses, there are 18 different hemagglutinin proteins (H1–H18) and 11 different neuraminidases (N1–N11) proteins. Their numbering is based on the order in which they were discovered. Any of the 18 H types and 11 N types can be the proteins on the outer membrane of a given influenza virus, but each virus has only one type of H and N. If you multiply 18×11 there is the potential for 198 different combinations of outer member H and N subtypes on influenza viruses, and many of these have been found in non-human animals, particularly birds. Influenza A H1N1 and/or H3N2 strains cause most of the disease in humans on a yearly basis. In some years, influenza B strains are the predominant cause of disease in humans. However, unlike influenza A strains, influenza B strains do not have this wide spectrum of hemagglutinins and neuraminidases, mutate more slowly, and do not cause global pandemics."

"That is very helpful. Before we get to my questions on avian influenza, I need to ask you about the epidemiology of annual influenza outbreaks. What percentage of the population is infected during non-pandemic years?"

"Each year, influenza viruses cause epidemics of disease where 5–10% of the population becomes infected with an influenza A and/or B virus. Non-tropical countries experience most of the cases in wintertime and hence the term 'seasonal influenza'. However, in tropical countries, the disease can occur periodically throughout the year. In the US, influenza illness results in 100,000–700,000 hospitalizations and 12,000 to 56,000 deaths depending on the severity of the disease in a given year. Globally, there are 3–5 million cases of severe influenza annually, resulting in 300,000 to 650,000 deaths each year."

"Wow. can someone be infected with the same virus strain more than once during their lifetime?"

"The hemagglutinin and neuraminidase proteins undergo genetic mutations on a frequent basis. This enables a particular strain, for example, an H1N1 strain, to change enough that a person can be infected by an H1N1 strain several times over their lifetime."

"Wow. Are these mutations the reason why flu vaccines are often less than 50% effective at preventing influenza disease?"

"It's one of the main reasons but it is important to note that the effectiveness of the vaccine is better at preventing severe flu disease, defined by the person requiring hospitalization or dying, than in preventing mild to moderate disease. These genetic changes cause us to make frequent changes to the influenza vaccine. The WHO Consultation of Influenza Viruses Vaccine for the Northern and Southern Hemisphere meet twice a year to determine if changes are required in the H1N1, H3N2 or B influenza strains in the vaccine. Once the Consultation group makes their recommendations, the vaccine companies begin the process to make the vaccine. Most companies still grow the influenza virus vaccine strains in chicken eggs and this entire process takes 5–6 months."

This last statement surprises David. "I thought most companies are now growing the virus in cell cultures and this allows the vaccine to be made in less time?"

"Approximately 90% of the global supply of vaccine is still made using the 50+-year-old egg technology. Some companies have built new manufacturing plants so they can switch to growing the virus in cells, but it still only decreases the production time by a few weeks."

"Is this why only about 10% of the vaccine used in the 2009 influenza pandemic made its way to low-income countries?"

"Great question. This is one of multiple reasons that decrease the impact of an influenza vaccine on an influenza pandemic. Let me give you some background information about influenza pandemics and this will help me answer your question.

"We know that multiple influenza pandemics have occurred every century. For a pandemic to happen, the virus's genetic makeup changes enough that most or all of the world's population have no immunity to the virus. An H1N1 influenza virus that originated in North American domestic or wild birds caused the 1918 influenza pandemic. This avian influenza virus mutated in a way that allowed the virus to infect about a third of the world's population. This pandemic resulted in 40 to 100 million deaths globally, including ~500,000 in the US. The 1918 pandemic is the deadliest event in recorded history, exceeding the number of deaths caused by other microbes, including smallpox, bubonic plague and HIV."

"Which influenza A strains have caused pandemics?"

"The three influenza virus strains that we know previously caused pandemics are H1N1, H2N2 and H3N2. The two major factors that determine how severe a pandemic will be are how easily the virus transmits between humans and how lethal the virus is. The cause of the 1918 and 2009 pandemic was an H1N1 virus containing avian genetic material and this caused tremendous concern that the 2009 pandemic could be as bad as the 1918 pandemic. While both viruses transmitted quickly throughout the global population, the lethality of the 1918 virus was much greater than the 2009 virus."

"Do we have any information to help us predict if another pandemic will occur?"

"The next influenza pandemic is a matter of when, not if, and we still don't have a good understanding regarding what genetic factors control transmissibility and lethality. Therefore, we can't predict when the next pandemic will occur or how severe it will be. Given what happened in the 1918 pandemic, many global health experts are particularly concerned about the risk that a more deadly avian flu virus will one day mutate in a way that allows the virus to infect and kill a large proportion of the global population."

"Can any influenza A strain cause a pandemic?"

"It's unclear. Since 1918, only viruses with H1, H2 and H3 hemagglutinin proteins have caused pandemics. Although the evidence is less certain, it appears this is also true for the earlier pandemics of 1831 and 1889. While the avian viruses H5N1 and H7N9 demonstrated that a person infected with one of these viruses has a high chance of death, it remains unclear if they will develop the ability to transmit between people at a high rate."

"Can you tell me more about the avian H5N1 and H7N9 outbreaks?"

"In the early 1990s, a bird H5N1 strain was killing poultry in very large numbers throughout Asia, North Africa and the Middle East. The first human case was detected in Guangdong, China, in 1996. Later on in Hong Kong in 1997, 18 humans were infected and six died. Since then, around 700 people have developed this disease with a death rate of around 60%. Almost all cases of H5N1 infection in people are associated with close contact with infected live or dead birds. The virus does not infect humans easily, and spread from person to person is rare. There is also no evidence that the disease can spread between people through properly prepared and thoroughly cooked food. Over the past few years, the number of human H5N1 cases is decreasing."

"That's good to hear. What about the H7N9 avian virus?"

"The H7N9 virus emerged in China in 2013 and to date has caused disease in over 750 people, killing   ~40% of them. Unlike H5N1, transmission between family members and between unrelated individuals has occurred. Furthermore, the spread of the virus from travelers coming from China to other countries has happened in a small number of cases. Given the pandemic potential of avian influenza A H7N9 and other novel influenza A viruses, it is crucial to continue to monitor and characterize these viruses."

"Would it be fair to say that the situation with avian influenza seems to be getting worse in the past several decades?"

"In the past century, in addition to the 1918 and 2009 pandemics, there have been two other influenza pandemics in 1957 and 1968. Each of these pandemics has been caused by a novel influenza A virus of avian and/or swine origin. During the past two decades, the number of reported infections caused by novel influenza A viruses has steadily increased, partly due to improved surveillance and diagnostic testing, but also due to overcrowding of people, poultry and pigs. The available virological, epidemiological and ecological information suggests that the H7N9 virus is the highest risk for emerging as a pandemic, among all evaluated novel influenza A viruses.

"I worked with the Chinese CDC on several occasions in the past and found them helpful. Have you been working with them?"

"I just came back from the Chinese CDC in Beijing two weeks ago. Based on what they learned from the H5N1 outbreak, they are now aggressively shutting open-air markets where H7N9-infected poultry exist. They are also in the process of developing an H7N9 vaccine for poultry to help contain the geographic spread of the virus."

"Thank you so much for the update. I see why the Director-General is so concerned about avian influenza. Do you have any good news I can share with her?"

"Overall, I believe the risk of an H5N1 pandemic is on the decline, and it is certainly possible the same thing will happen to the current H7N9 outbreak in Asia. The bad news is that future mutations could change all of that. We don't know how this story is going to end. The cost of a major influenza outbreak will far outweigh the price of prevention. All of us in public health must remain vigilant. David, do you mind if I ask you a few questions?"

"Fire away."

"The WHO previously published pandemic preparedness guidance in 1999 and an updated version in 2005. The 2009 pandemic had very little vaccine available during the first six months for any country, but once the vaccine started rolling out of the manufacturing plants, over 90% went to high-income countries. Why did that happen and what needs to happen to fix this situation?"

"Richard, that is a great question. The WHO has been trying for years to find an equitable way to have the wealthier countries share resources with developing countries during an influenza pandemic. High-income and middle-income countries in the Pan American region have contracts with vaccine manufacturers to buy the influenza vaccine every year. During the 2009 pandemic, the WHO was able to get a commitment from some companies for 10% of the influenza vaccine they produce. A similar situation existed for Tamiflu, the only drug available for treating influenza throughout the globe. Since then, the WHO has worked hard to try to ensure sufficient quantities of vaccines and drugs would be available for low- and middle-income countries during a future pandemic."

"Do you think this is an obtainable goal?"

"Not at this time," David bluntly replies.

"I had a feeling that was the case. Since epidemic influenza kills many people each year, what are the major reasons that impede the annual use of the flu vaccine in low- and middle-income countries?"

"The cost of the vaccine and lack of an infrastructure to deliver the vaccine to children and adults on a yearly basis are two of the most important reasons. In many of the lowest income countries, the amount of money governments spend on healthcare is very small and most of it goes towards treatment rather than prevention. While the health ministers in these countries support the use of vaccines, the money available to buy vaccines used outside of those routinely given to children less than 5 years old is sparse. The Global Alliance for Vaccines and Immunization (Gavi) helps these countries pay for vaccines, but the large number of recommended routine childhood vaccines still result in many countries prioritizing the ones they use. Outside the Region of the Americas, very few low- and middle-income countries have added influenza vaccine into their routine immunization program."

"How much progress has been made by the WHO to ensure that low- and middle-income countries get access to influenza vaccines in a pandemic?"

"The progress is slow. Vaccine companies are currently producing about 1.5 billion doses of influenza vaccine each year. They are not going to build the manufacturing capacity to make the 7-plus billion vaccine doses needed for a pandemic unless this quantity of vaccine is purchased on an annual basis for epidemic influenza. Development of a vaccine that would protect against all influenza A viruses is probably the best long-term answer."

Richard nods but voices his concern about when this type of vaccine will be available. "I agree, but I don't think we are likely to have the so-called 'universal' influenza vaccine anytime soon. I would love to continue this conversation at dinner tomorrow, but for now, I have to head home and I also suspect you must be tired after your travel from Geneva and a long afternoon here. Do you want me to drop you off at the hotel before I head home?"

"It's definitely been a long day, but so informative. Thank you again for showing me around the facilities. I will walk to the hotel since it is only a few minutes away and I need to stretch my legs. I look forward to continuing our discussion at dinner tomorrow."

Melinda escorts David to the CDC entrance where he picks up his passport. When he gets to the hotel, he orders room service and after eating, he quickly falls asleep. In the middle of the night, he wakes up in a cold sweat from a dream where the H7N9 avian influenza has mutated in a way that allows easy transmission of the virus between people. The virus is spreading across the world and killing half of those who are infected. He lays awake the rest of the night thinking about what can be done to prevent this nightmare from becoming reality.

Chapter 8

Centers for Disease Control and Prevention Atlanta, US, November 2016, Day 2

The following morning Melinda meets David at the security entrance and escorts him to Elena Sanchez's office. When he arrives at the office, Elena is standing outside the door, dressed in the navy-blue public health uniform worn by many of the CDC staff.

"Thanks so much for taking the time to meet with me. Yesterday, you were not wearing your public health uniform, but today you are. Is this required when you are meeting people from outside of the CDC?"

"Most of us wear the uniform when meeting with outside people, but it is not a requirement. Does the WHO have a uniform requirement?"

"Not that I know about. If it does, I have been violating the rule for decades."

Elena laughs. "Can I get you some coffee or tea before we talk about the Zika virus?"

"No, thanks. I filled the caffeine tank at breakfast. I just spent two weeks in Brazil at the Director-General's request and have a lot of questions about the Zika outbreak in the Americas that I hope you will be able to answer."

"I am not sure there are many answers at this point, but I will do my best."

"When I was in Brazil, they told me that the Zika virus infections are now being seen on the US mainland. What have you been seeing?"

"Prior to 2014, we saw a few cases in the United States (US), all of whom had traveled to regions where the Zika virus was known to exist. From 2015 through to 2016, large outbreaks of the Zika virus occurred in the Americas, resulting in an increase in travel-associated cases in the US. We also saw widespread transmission in the US Territories of Puerto Rico and the Virgin Islands. Recently, we have seen limited local transmission in Florida and Texas."

"How many cases have you seen on the US mainland, Puerto Rico and the Virgin Islands?"

"In 2016, the CDC made the Zika virus a nationally notifiable disease. To date, in the US mainland, there have been over 5,000 symptomatic Zika virus cases reported. Most of these cases are in travelers returning from affected areas, but over 200 cases occurred through presumed local mosquito-borne transmission mainly in southern Florida, but also in southern Texas. Some of the cases occurred through sexual transmission from a partner who had traveled outside the country. In the US Territories, there have been more than 37,000 reported Zika virus cases, with the great majority due to local mosquito-borne transmission. There appear to be cases of congenital Zika virus infection where the fetus is infected while in the mother's womb, but confirmation of these cases needs further laboratory and medical imaging data."

"I didn't realize the number of cases in the US and its territories was this large. How are you trying to control the local transmission and decrease the number of travel cases?"

"We're taking a multi-prong approach including putting out educational material for the public about the risk of travel and noting that pregnant women should not travel to any place where the Zika virus disease is endemic. For women and their partners who are considering having a child, they should also avoid travel to these areas. When this is not possible, then the women should avoid becoming pregnant for at least six months after their travel has ended, since we know the Zika virus can be present in men's semen for months after they become infected. Another point we are emphasizing is that anyone traveling should stay in places where there are window screens and use mosquito spray when outside. We make it clear that those who don't get sick while traveling could still be infected with the virus since most cases are asymptomatic."

"Has this been effective in decreasing travel of pregnant women and their partners?"

'We hope so, but won't know for at least a year. We just finished a phone survey showing that the majority of women who are pregnant have decided to postpone their travels. For those who have partners who traveled to infected areas, most are using condoms during sex. On the other hand, the survey suggests less than half of those who are considering getting pregnant are postponing their travels, but intend to follow our other precautions. A more definitive answer to your question won't be available until we get a few years down the road and see whether there is a decrease in the number of infants with congenital Zika virus disease being born to women who traveled to endemic areas."

"I read somewhere that you are spraying for mosquitoes. How are you deciding what areas in the US and its territories to spray?"

"We're trapping mosquitoes in various areas in southern Florida and Texas and testing them for the Zika virus. We then selectively use planes to spray the areas where the virus-infected mosquitoes exist. We're using more widespread spraying in Puerto Rico and the Virgin Islands because it is clear there are virus-infected mosquitoes throughout these two territories."

"Are people living in the areas being sprayed expressing concern about the chemicals in the spray?"

"Before spraying, we have done a lot of public education about why and where we're spraying and there has been minimal pushback."

"I saw a few infants born with congenital Zika infections and microcephaly while I was in Brazil, but I wonder if you can give me a better idea of the full spectrum of the disease?"

"The various manifestations of the congenital infection are still being elucidated, but it is clear that the main impact is on the neurologic system and this can occur even when the head size is normal. Some babies demonstrate a substantial delay in both motor and communications skills. The specific defects may depend on the timing of the infection during pregnancy, but unlike rubella virus, the Zika virus can cause damage anytime during pregnancy. We are doing several studies to determine the extent of the abnormalities that occur and when this happens during pregnancy."

"Do we know how often a congenital disease occurs in pregnant women infected with the virus?"

"While the initial data from Brazil suggested the incidence of congenital infection was as high as 50%, more recent data suggests that the infection rate is around 7%. We are working on developing tests that can definitively differentiate Zika virus infection from dengue and chikungunya infections, which will allow us to better define the impact of timing of the infection with the types of congenital abnormalities that can occur."

"Where do things stand with the development of drugs and vaccines for the Zika virus?"

"The US National Institutes of Health and other groups are working on developing drugs and vaccines, both internally and through funding grant proposals from academic researchers. I don't think drugs are the answer to preventing congenital Zika virus since so many people, including pregnant women, are asymptomatic when infected by the virus. We are involved with planning studies to evaluate vaccines as they become available and may be doing one in Brazil within the next few months."

"When I was down in Brazil, I actually got to visit with the group planning to conduct that study. They hope to be doing this vaccine study in the next few months. Do you think this timeframe is possible?"

"I'm not sure. The number of Zika cases has decreased dramatically over the last two months. We are not sure of the reasons for this decrease since it is summer in Brazil and the mosquito population is at full force. If the outbreak is truly resolving, we will not be able to determine if the vaccine is efficacious."

"I spent a fair amount of time with Venetia Sousa, one of the investigators on the project. Do you know her?"

"She is a friend of mine. I just spoke with her a few days ago and their group is beginning to realize we may not be able to do the vaccine trial until another Zika virus outbreak occurs."

"When I met with Venetia this past September, she was in the second trimester of her pregnancy and was going to her doctor for Zika virus testing. Do you know what the test results showed?"

"The blood test came back positive. She is concerned about the test result, but is aware this could also be due to several other viruses that are endemic in Brazil. She also had an ultrasound done and they didn't see any abnormalities in her baby that suggested congenital Zika virus infection. This made her feel better, but she is aware that some fetuses with congenital Zika virus don't show any manifestations until after they are born."

"I'm sorry to hear that her test came back positive. It must be hard to live with that uncertainty. Do you know when her due date is?"

"Early next year. Venetia told me her husband, Luiz, has supported her throughout her pregnancy and they both find strength through their religion."

"I will send her an email tonight to let her know I am thinking about them."

Elena and David continue to discuss various aspects of the Zika virus outbreak. When they are finished, she walks with David over to the CDC Global Division where he spends the rest of the day in various meetings and catching up with several friends who work there.

***

David leaves the CDC campus around 5:30 p.m. and walks across the street to the Emory Conference center hotel where he is staying. He decides he has enough time to take a quick nap and shower before meeting Richard at the hotel. He enters The Club Room restaurant at 7 p.m. and sees Richard already sitting at a table. They take a few minutes to look over the menu. Richard orders a grilled Scottish salmon while David gets the braised short rib. David then starts the conversation by asking Richard what made him decide to go into public health.

"I was born in New York City in 1972 and lived there for the first 30 years of my life. Just before graduating from high school, my mother died of bacterial pneumonia after an influenza infection. After taking a year off from school, I decided I wanted to become a physician. I stayed in New York because I thought my father needed me there and so I went to college and medical school at Columbia University. I did an internal medicine residency and infectious disease fellowship at New York University's Bellevue Hospital and then went back to Columbia to obtain a Master's degree in Public Health. Thereafter, I left New York to go to Atlanta to complete a two-year CDC Epidemic Intelligence Service Officer training program. Upon finishing this program, I accepted a full-time position at the CDC working in the Influenza Division. Since then I have filled up several passports traveling to many countries chasing the ever-evolving influenza virus."

"You sound like you travel as much as I do. Does your work consume all your time or do you have a family?"

"I got married ten years ago. My wife is a pediatrician and my daughter is seven years old. How about you?"

"I've never been married, but I am dating someone who works for Médecins Sans Frontières. Your story gives me hope it might not be too late to start a family."

"I highly recommend marriage. My wife and child keep me grounded and give me a life outside of work."

"Did your wife want you to take the CDC Interim-Director position?"

"We had several long discussions about this. Both of us are very close with the previous CDC Director and his wife. The week after he announced his resignation, we had dinner with them. He felt I was the best person to take on this job. Later that night, my wife suggested I should at least temporally take on the Acting Director position and we would see how it worked out."

"Interesting that you had this conversation with your wife. I had a similar conversation with Aceline, the woman I'm dating, when I accepted my new position as Interim-Deputy Director of the Human Emergencies Program. Besides the increased time commitment of the position, what were your other concerns?"

"Where do I start? The previous CDC Director resigned in large part due to the recent election results. During the last five decades, every time there was a Presidential election that resulted in the Republican Party controlling the White House and Congress, the CDC budget underwent major cuts. Many of the President-elect's comments during the election campaign suggest he holds science in low regard. Since winning the election, he has indicated that the budget he submits to Congress will request a 20% budget cut for the CDC. I don't think Congress will go along with this type of draconian cut, but any cut will impact our ability to respond to new outbreaks in the US and across the globe."

"The WHO Director-General has also expressed a similar concern after the President announced he was considering decreasing the US commitment to global funding in developing countries. What do you think can be done about this?"

"Many of us are already working with members of Congress who support the CDC and other science-based agencies. Based on various conversations, I think we can head off most of the cuts, but the proof of this will come next year."

"What are the President's views on vaccines?"

"He thinks vaccines are unsafe. In 2014, he wrote a tweet suggesting the number of vaccines given to infants was contributing to rising autism rates. During his presidential campaign, he met with prominent anti-vaccination figures, including Andrew Wakefield, who published a paper containing falsified data and used it to claim that the measles component of the MMR vaccine was causing autism. He also met with Robert Kennedy Jr., a well-known opponent of vaccines, and reportedly asked him to head a vaccine safety board he wants to establish."

David is incredulous. "You must be kidding."

"Sadly, I am not."

"Knowing all this, would you still consider taking the permanent CDC Director position if offered to you?"

"My wife asked me the same question last night and I told her I didn't know. A lot will depend on what happens with the CDC budget and who becomes the Secretary of Health. Dealing with the threat of budget cuts seems to be the main trigger for my migraine headaches."

"That's not good. Is there a leading candidate for the Secretary of Health position that might help you deal with the threat of budget cuts?"

"There have been half a dozen names mentioned, but no clear top choice."

Their entrees arrive at their table along with red wine. David takes a few minutes to process what he is hearing.

"It appears I will not have any good news for the Director-General on the political side, but maybe there is some better news around preparing for the next influenza pandemic. Could we discuss what you think the critical components of being better prepared for the next influenza pandemic will be?"

"Sure."

"Yesterday I mentioned the possibility of a universal influenza vaccine. How far along are the National Institutes of Health and other groups in developing a vaccine that can protect against all influenza A strains?"

"To be candid, not close. For years, there has been a lot of chatter but little progress in making a universal influenza vaccine that protects against all, or at least most, strains of influenza. The virus is a chameleon that frequently changes its genetic makeup. This allows the virus to thrive. Over the next five years, it is conceivable there will be incremental progress that improves the effectiveness of an influenza vaccine. However, the development of the so-called "universal vaccine" that can protect against a major genetic shift that allows a strain to cause a pandemic is likely at least a decade away."

"What is needed to move that process along faster?"

"Many researchers believe we need to create a broader research portfolio that would allow us to better understand the immunologic response in humans the first time they are infected with an influenza virus and how this impacts the immune response to subsequent influenza viruses. Even with that knowledge, it is still more likely there will be incremental improvements in developing a more effective vaccine than creating a vaccine that protects against all strains of influenza viruses. Doing this type of research will take a lot more money than is currently available, unfortunately."

"In addition to the virus characteristics that increase disease severity and cause higher mortality, are there also human factors that increase the risk of developing a severe disease?"

"There is increasing evidence some people are genetically susceptible to more severe disease. Additionally, people with chronic conditions, including heart and lung disease, are more at risk for severe disease. During the last decade, we have determined that obesity is another important risk factor and the incidence of obesity is increasing in many countries."

"Besides creating a better influenza vaccine, what else can we do to decrease deaths before the next influenza pandemic?"

"Most of the deaths due to seasonal and pandemic influenza are due to secondary bacterial pneumonias. The two most common bacteria causing these pneumonias are *Streptococcus pneumoniae* and *Staphylococcus aureus*. We now have a reasonably effective vaccine against the pneumococcus, but need one against Staph aureus. Several companies have been working on developing this vaccine for the past decade, but to date, none has proven effective."

"What about drugs to treat influenza?"

"Tamiflu is a reasonably effective drug against influenza viruses. However, during the 2009 influenza pandemic, there was not enough of the drug available. We are working with the WHO and other organizations to try to increase the supply of Tamiflu. However, in a pandemic situation, it is unlikely that we would have enough drugs to give to everyone who needs it."

"What about new drugs against influenza?"

"Several companies are working on new drugs against influenza and I expect at least one of these will be available in a few years."

David notices Richard looking at his watch. "I really appreciate the information you shared with me. I know you would like to get home to be with your family."

"Are you flying back to Geneva tomorrow?"

"Yes. I enjoyed meeting you. Please feel free to call me if things come up where I can be of help."

"Same here and I appreciate the offer of a direct line into the WHO."

When David is back in his room, he calls Aceline to see if she can spend the holiday season with him. Aceline indicates she had already worked it out to spend Christmas weekend with her parents in France, and will then come to join him in Geneva for at least a week. David tells her he is counting the days until they are together.

Chapter 9

Geneva, Switzerland
Winter of 2016–17

D avid meets with the Director-General the following week to update her on the ongoing Zika virus outbreak in the Americas and the status of the avian influenza outbreak in Asia. She thanks David for the information and expresses her deep concern about the expanding number of outbreaks during the 21st century. She asks David to work with his Health Emergencies group over the next few months to strengthen the current plan to deal with this issue.

David meets with Philippe Bernard, the Associate Director of the WHO Health Emergencies Division, that afternoon. "I just updated the Director-General on what I learned during my trip to the CDC. She is very concerned about the four-fold increase in outbreaks during the last few decades and wants to enhance our current Human Emergencies Strategy Plan to decrease the frequency and severity of these outbreaks. I need you to update me on the status of all of the current global outbreaks. My current list includes the following diseases:

1) Yellow fever virus in Africa and the Americas,
2) Dengue virus in Asia, Africa and the Americas,
3) Chikungunya virus in Africa and the Americas,
4) Hepatitis E virus in Africa and Asia,

5) Lassa fever virus in Africa, the Americas and Europe,
6) Ebola virus in Africa, and
7) The mutated strain of coronavirus causing a new disease, the Middle East Respiratory Syndrome in Saudi Arabia, Qatar and the United Arab Emirates."

"Am I missing anything?"

Philippe sighs. "Unfortunately, yes. A recent cholera outbreak in the Western Horn of Africa, including Ethiopia, Somalia and Yemen. This outbreak has the potential to be really bad."

"Tell me more about what makes you think this cholera outbreak could be worse than others we have dealt with in the past."

"The first wave of this new cholera outbreak was causing moderately severe diarrhea and dehydration. The humanitarian healthcare agencies working in those countries were able to provide rehydration fluids, antibiotics and other supportive care to everyone seeking help and the mortality rate remained below 1%. However, in the last few months, a second wave of cholera is spreading rapidly across the Western Horn of Africa with a greater mortality rate. To date, there are more than 70,000 cases and 1,400 deaths."

"Do we know why the mortality rate is higher than usual?"

"We are part of an ongoing on-site investigation to determine whether the cholera strain causing this outbreak has become more virulent or resistant to the antibiotics being used. I think it's more likely that the ongoing severe drought and food shortages occurring in this area are the main factors making the outbreak worse. Somalia and Yemen also contain areas that are hard for humanitarian groups to work in due to armed conflicts. In Yemen, the cholera response is happening on top of prolonged fighting between the government and rebel forces. This war has already destroyed most of the country's infrastructure including many healthcare facilities, and most of the healthcare personnel who are still working there have gone without pay for a long time. In Somalia, the drought has caused food shortages in 75% of the country and a lack of clean drinking water. Recently, the cholera epidemic in that area of Africa has spread into the region of Ethiopia that borders Somalia. Médecins Sans

Frontières and other humanitarian agencies are responding differently in each country based on the specific underlying issues."

"Are the humanitarian groups able to cope?"

"The number of confirmed or suspected cases has doubled since the start of the outbreak and spread into new areas in these countries. The humanitarian groups are expanding their efforts and sometimes pulling resources from other places. When possible, they work on improving access to clean water and educating the local population on how to limit transmission. There are still huge gaps in the responses."

"Where do things stand with using the cholera vaccine? Does the Global Alliance for Vaccines and Immunization (Gavi) have enough doses in their stockpile to enable us to stop the outbreak?"

"More than one million people living in high-risk areas received the two-dose oral vaccine so far. We are working with Gavi and the cholera vaccine manufacturers to increase the supply."

David's frustration is increasing by the moment. "Sometimes I feel that all we do is chase our tail around in a circle. The current Human Emergencies Strategy Plan is not getting the job done and we need to think outside the paradigm proposed in the current plan. Before most of our group takes off for the holidays, we need to create a list of the major issues leading to these outbreaks and start working on potential new solutions that could substantially limit their frequency and severity. I want solutions that will get us beyond responding to each outbreak one at a time and find answers that will help us prevent these outbreaks from occurring."

"Some solutions will likely have a large price tag and based on previous history, I fear the major donors will not put more money on the table."

"We can work with healthcare economists to make the case that the cost of doing what is necessary to prevent these outbreaks is a lot less than the continuously increasing cost of responding to all of these major outbreaks. I know the Director-General believes this and will work tirelessly to find the additional funding."

"I will talk to the other members of our group before we hold our first meeting next week."

***

The following Monday, David meets with 12 members of his group that are not away on assignment. They discuss the various outbreaks that occurred during the past decade and what new solutions they would propose to limit their frequency and severity going forward. An intense, and at times heated, discussion lasts into the early evening. David thinks he has heard enough.

"It's getting late and I need to let you get home. This discussion has generated many new ideas. At this point, I would like us to concentrate on the following ones:

1) The use of new technologies to help make vaccines and drugs more accessible and easier to use during outbreaks.
2) The use of new technologies to improve sanitation in areas with frequent enteric disease outbreaks such as cholera and typhoid.
3) Genetic manipulation of mosquitoes to decrease their numbers.
4) Making better use of the knowledge of social scientists, including anthropologists, to better understand and interact with the various populations impacted by these outbreaks.

While many of the other ideas expressed today are good, I have chosen these four proposed solutions because we could potentially implement them within the next several years. Since there are 12 of you who are currently in town working on this issue, I would ask you to split up into groups of three based on your specific expertise. I need you to answer the following questions regarding how the proposed solution would affect outbreaks:

1) What will be the anticipated impact on mortality?
2) Will the frequency of outbreaks decrease and, if so, by how much?
3) Can the proposal affect more than one type of disease outbreak and, if so, which ones?
4) How long will it take until we can implement the proposed solution?
5) What is the estimated additional funding needed?

I realize this is a lot of work and all of you are going to be out of the office during part or all of the holiday season. I would propose we set up another meeting in the middle of January and see where things stand with each proposed solution. In the interim, please contact Philippe or me with any questions or concerns. One of us will be in town throughout the holidays and I will send you our holiday schedule by the end of the week."

***

David spends the rest of the week further considering the four potential solutions and how they could be refined and prioritized. The Christmas weekend comes and goes and finally, Aceline is arriving in Geneva that day. He sees she will be landing soon so he leaves to pick her up at the airport. He recognizes how excited he is to see her as he waits for her to come through Passport Control to the baggage area. He now realizes he was so consumed with work the past few weeks, he never asked her what she would like to do while they are together in Switzerland. While contemplating how to deal with his oversight, Aceline comes through the door. David wraps his arms around her and holds her tight for what seems like a long time.

"Thanks for picking me up and the warm embrace is a wonderful greeting."

"I can't tell you how much I missed you."

"Sure you can, and I would love to hear it."

David smirks. He has grown to appreciate Aceline's sense of humor and has, in fact, missed it. "I'll be happy to do so over dinner. However, first, I need to apologize for not asking you what you wanted to do while we are together this week."

"Apology accepted. Could we spend a few days in the Alps and the rest of the time in Geneva?"

"It may be hard to find an available hotel room in the Alps this time of year, but I might be able to pull a few strings."

"That would be great. Can we go to your apartment before we go to dinner?"

"Absolutely."

David's apartment is in the old town part of Geneva whose history goes back to 58 B.C. To get to his apartment, they drive through a labyrinth of small streets and picturesque squares filled with churches, cafés, restaurants, galleries and museums lined by historical buildings adorned with beautiful masonry façades. They arrive at his apartment and David carries Aceline's luggage up to the apartment.

"I have been to Geneva on two occasions, but never to this part of town. Can we go to dinner somewhere around here tonight and explore the area?"

"Would you like to take a nap before we go out to dinner?"

"Just a short one. Would it be possible for us to walk to the restaurant so I can see more of the city?"

"Can do."

An hour later, they start walking to the restaurant. Aceline notices the square has rows of lamps decorated with Christmas lights. They pass St. Peter's Cathedral and David suggests climbing the 157 steps up the north tower to take in the incredible views of the city and the lake. He notes that the cathedral was built in the 12th century on the site of an ancient Roman Temple from the 4th century. The original architecture was of a Romanesque style and it was the place where John Calvin preached Protestantism in the 16th century. Now, the cathedral displays a fusion of different styles with a neoclassical façade and an austere interior.

They walk past the Maison Tavel, the museum of Geneva's history, and onto the Place du Bourg-de-Four Square that is in the center of Geneva's Old Town where the Roman marketplace used to be. The middle of the square contains simple marble medieval fountains and many shops and restaurants. They finally arrive at the Café de Bourg-de-Four restaurant where David made a dinner reservation. This restaurant is small with a medieval atmosphere. Many nights, people dine outside so they can appreciate the unique history and atmosphere of the area. However, it is too cold tonight and they go inside. The owner of the restaurant knows David and takes them to a table for two, next to a window so that they can look outside.

"Aceline, the restaurant has some great Swiss food. I hope you like it."

"This looks like a perfect start to what I know will be a great week together."

"I texted my friend and he was able to get us a hotel room up in the Alps for three days. Do you like to ski?"

"Wow! You really were able to pull some strings. I love skiing and hiking in the mountains. This vacation with you is getting better by the minute."

"Ha, I do what I can. How was your visit with your family?"

"It was good, but during the last few times I visited, I could tell they were starting to feel their age. My mom has arthritis that is starting to limit her mobility, and her physician started her on a new medication. She and my dad are now back to taking the long walks they both enjoy. My dad was just diagnosed with prostate cancer and will be seeing a surgeon after the holidays to discuss the possibility of having his prostate removed."

"I am really sorry to hear that. I've heard prostate cancer is a slow-growing tumor and people often live more than 15 years, even without surgery or radiation therapy. How old is he?"

Aceline replies, "Both my parents are in their mid-60s. The time course is one of the issues my dad will be discussing with the surgeon."

"How is he coping with the news?

"He is anxious to hear what the doctor says, but otherwise seems to be dealing with it well."

"How are you feeling about it?

"I am okay. I am trying to put off getting too worried until we hear back about his prognosis. On a different note, I am curious to know what you would have done during this holiday if I wasn't with you."

"Probably working. The Director-General is very concerned with the increasing number of infectious disease global outbreaks and asked me to come up with additional approaches that will lead to less frequent and severe outbreaks."

"Do you need to work while I am here?"

"There's always work to do. However, while you are here, my full attention will be on you and only you. When I saw you come through the door at the airport, I was so excited that my heart started racing."

"Until we started dating, I thought you were clueless about what a woman feels and needs. All I can say is I was wrong. There is a lot of romance in your soul. Speaking of which, I know our relationship has moved along rapidly and I am curious about what you were thinking about what all of this means."

David looks a little flustered. "I mean, I don't want to see anyone else. I really like you and am enjoying seeing where this is going. What were you thinking?"

Aceline smiles. "Oh, in my free time I've been on loads of other dates."

David lets out a nervous laugh.

Aceline grabs his hand. "I am totally kidding. I feel the exact same way. I've been nothing but happy since we went to Casablanca together."

David lets out a sigh of relief, laughs and looks into Aceline's eyes. "I am so happy to hear that."

The waiter comes over and takes David's and Aceline's orders, which include a Caesar salad, chicken diablo, mussels and red wine. They spend the next two hours enjoying their meal and each other. After dinner, they walk back to David's apartment, and once there, Aceline takes a small package out of her suitcase. "While I was with my parents, I had a chance to buy something for you."

"I feel bad that I didn't get something for you."

"I did not buy you a gift expecting something in return. Please open it."

David opens the package and pulls out a watch, "Wow, this watch is beautiful. I don't know how to thank you."

"Come to bed and I'm sure we can figure something out."

***

Over the next four days, David and Aceline spend their time wandering around Geneva and enjoying each other's company. The following day they take a four-hour train ride up to the Omnia, a 5-star hotel that is within walking distance of the closest gondola lift and the Gornergrat alpine railway where they can take the 13 km ride to the Matterhorn. During the daytime, they spend time skiing and hiking in the Alps and the nights dining in various restaurants. On the return train ride back to Geneva, they are both quiet as they realize their vacation is almost over.

When they approach the train station, David looks over at Aceline and notices she is staring at him.

"Aceline, I can't believe this is our last night together before you go back to the DRC. I was thinking rather than going out to dinner tonight I could cook at home. Are you okay with that?"

"Sounds perfect. Do you want to stop at the market on our way home?"

"Why don't you head back to the apartment and take a nap while I go shopping. I will wake you up when dinner is ready."

"That is a deal I can't pass up."

As they get near the apartment, David heads off to go food shopping, but first stops off at another store to buy a gift for Aceline. He then buys the food he needs for their dinner and heads back to the apartment where Aceline is asleep. He prepares dinner and pours the wine before he wakes her.

"Time to get up, sleepyhead."

"What time is it?

"7:30 p.m."

"Oh wow. I slept for more than two hours. Whatever you are making sure smells good."

"Cheese and fruit crepes. I hope you like it."

"We shall see how good your culinary skills are."

"Since it is too expensive to eat out every night in Geneva, I think my years of bachelorhood have turned me into a fairly good cook."

Aceline is impressed with the dinner and when they finish she offers to clean up.

"I'll take you up on your offer, but first I want to give you a gift. I need to preface this by saying you were right when you said your initial impression of me was that I had no clue about what a woman thinks or wants."

"Hold on. After I said that, I did note I was wrong."

"Well, we are about to find out if you are correct. This past week has been wonderful. I have been skiing many times up in the Alps and I have always appreciated the majesty of skiing down those beautiful mountains. However, every time we skied or hiked in the mountains, all I could think about was you. I've never felt this way before."

David gets on his knees and opens the box. "Aceline, I know I love you. Though we've only been dating for a few months, we've known each other for several years, and I am sure you are the person I want to live with for the rest of my life. Will you marry me?"

Aceline's facial expression is one of shock, and David is unsure what this means. He starts to get nervous when finally Aceline says, "Yes! I thought I was falling in love with you even before you left Africa the last time, and after our time in Casablanca, the feeling was bursting within me. I knew from the way you looked at me and touched me that you also loved me, but I didn't know how long it would take you to figure out."

David chuckles. "Not as dense as I appear, huh?"

Aceline smiles as she puts the ring on her finger. "You always surprise me. The ring is beautiful."

"The owner of the jewelry store is a friend of mine and she helped me to pick it out. I'm glad you like it."

"I love it. We can talk more about all of this later, but right now we need to put the rest of the night to good use."

"One of the many reasons why I love you."

David drives Aceline to the airport the following morning. He tells Aceline he promised the Director-General he would give her an expanded Emergency Outbreak Plan by the end of March. Aceline shares that she still has over a week of vacation time left before July and would be happy to spend the remaining time with him in Geneva.

Chapter 10

Geneva Switzerland, Spring of 2017

David and his group meet frequently during the next three months to develop the Human Emergencies Strategy Plan they started before the holidays. They discuss each of the options in detail and rank them based on impact and cost. The one getting the highest priority is the use of new technologies to improve sanitation in areas with frequent outbreaks of enteric gastrointestinal diseases. During this time, the Gates Foundation created a competition "Reinvent the Toilet Challenge" in an effort to develop "next-generation" toilets that could deliver safe and sustainable sanitation to lower-income countries. Multiple universities participated in this competition and the California Institute of Technology received the $100,000 first-place award for designing a solar-powered toilet that generates hydrogen and electricity. Loughborough University in the United Kingdom won the $60,000 second-place award for a toilet that produces biological charcoal, minerals and clean water. The group felt these technologies would be effective for decreasing the frequency and severity of many enteric diseases causing severe diarrhea, including cholera and typhoid. Additionally, the technology could be available within the next couple of years and the anticipated cost would be low enough for donors to fund it.

The proposal to increase the use of anthropologists and other social scientists to help the WHO better understand how to effectively communicate and interact with the various populations impacted by these outbreaks obtained the second-highest priority. David had never interacted with an anthropologist prior to the 2014 Ebola outbreak in Western Africa. During that outbreak, several anthropologists with expertise in the cultural traditions of different Western African ethnic groups proved crucial to effectively communicate with the different populations within Western Africa. Based on this experience and the more recent one in the DRC where the anthropologist, Kamanda Mutombo, helped them write the consent forms for those being vaccinated with a reduced doses of the yellow fever vaccine, David and his group felt anthropologists would be very helpful in many different types of outbreaks that involved marginalized populations. Additionally, the anthropologists could help the WHO better implement programs that could prevent or more effectively intervene in outbreaks, such as the use of the yellow fever vaccine in the routine childhood immunization program. The use of anthropologists for these types of activities could start immediately and the cost would be lower than the other proposals.

The proposal to use genetic manipulation techniques to decrease the mosquito population is high risk and high reward. During the past two decades, more than 100 countries have experienced outbreaks from diseases carried by Aedes mosquitoes. These outbreaks involved dengue, chikungunya, yellow fever, and Zika viruses. Global warming is increasing the geographical spread of the Aedes mosquito. If the genetic manipulation of mosquitoes proved successful in decreasing the number of mosquitoes, it would likely decrease the incidence of these viral diseases and do the same for malaria caused by Anopheles mosquitoes. The major concern with this proposal was that previous attempts to control mosquito populations using other techniques had been ongoing for many years with only modest success. They suggested awaiting the results of several ongoing mosquito genetic manipulation studies, including the one in Brazil, before adding this to the plan.

The development of one or more new technologies to make vaccines and drugs easier to administer to people would be helpful for most, if not all, outbreaks, including pandemics. However, these new technologies are at least five years away from receiving regulatory approval. The group suggested the WHO, along with Gavi, consider forming a group of independent experts to consider ways to speed this process up.

***

David meets with the Director-General in the last week of March. He presents each of the four proposals and the rationale for how they prioritized the top two.

"David, I think the group has undergone a thoughtful analysis of what can be done to lessen the frequency and severity of infectious disease outbreaks. I support your recommendations and will now pursue additional monies to fund the two highest rated proposals. However, I need to remind you that the Director-General position is limited to ten years and my time in this position will end in a few months. The World Health Assembly, is the governing body of the WHO is composed of Health Ministers from 194 countries. It will select the next person for the Director-General position in May 2017. The new Director-General's ideas on what needs to occur to stop these outbreaks may be different than mine."

"I understand. While I know you will not be leaving for several months, I want to let you know how much I enjoyed working with you and greatly appreciate all the support you have given me."

"Thank you, David, and I have also liked working with you. Please let your group know that I value the work they are doing. I would appreciate it if you could send me the full written report of the Human Emergencies Strategy Plan as soon as possible."

"Will do."

***

David works on the written report the following week. He finds the report is taking him longer than usual because his thoughts keep drifting to Aceline who is arriving at the Geneva airport later today. He finally emails the Director-General the document and heads to the airport. Aceline gives him a big smile when she sees him and he embraces her. On the drive back to his apartment, they pass near the WHO headquarters.

"David, I've never been to the WHO headquarters. Would it be possible for me to go inside with you sometime?"

"Of course. Do you want to go now?"

"I have something else in mind. Let's first go back to the apartment." David gives her a quizzical look.

"David, the look on your face is precious. It has been a long time since I've been with a man and I miss the intimacy. Now, when we are apart, I miss it even more."

"I was hoping that was what you meant. This afternoon we can go to the Botanical Gardens and eat lunch there. After, we can go up to WHO headquarters."

"It would be great if we can walk there since the weather is wonderful. I could also use the exercise after sitting on the plane for what seemed like forever."

"Walking works for me."

Later that afternoon, David and Aceline stroll along Lake Geneva toward the Botanical Gardens. He remembers she told him that she had been in Geneva a couple of times. "How well do you know Geneva?"

"My parents took me here once when I was a child, once with my ex for two days and when I came to visit you a few months ago. Anything you tell me is likely to be new to me."

"Aceline, your tour guide, David, is at your beckon call. You will get to experience a much different Geneva in the spring than you did in the winter. I have been wondering for a while why you usually call your former husband your 'ex' rather than by his name?"

"The man cheated on me and then lied about it. It took several years to get over it and during that time, I mostly referred to him as my ex. I hope to never have to go through that again."

David squeezes her hand. "Aceline, I feel certain you will not. I adore everything about you. I've never felt this way before. I never cheated on my two former girlfriends and my feelings for them were much less intense than those I have for you."

Aceline stops walking along the shoreline and in the middle of a crowd of people gives David a long soulful kiss. "I think about you every waking hour of the day and you are in my dreams every night. Now I am ready for you to be my tour guide."

David puts his arm around her shoulder. "Alright, the tour starts now. Lake Geneva is the largest body of water in Switzerland, and is larger than all other lakes connected with the main valleys of the Alps. The lake is crescent-shaped with the city of Geneva on the western end and the town of Montreux on the eastern end. The northern side of the lake is opposite from where we are standing and is 95 km long and the southern shore is 72 km in length. The greatest depth of the lake is 310 m and the bottom of the lake is 62 m above sea level. I often walk home from the WHO and sometimes take a small detour so I can walk along the lake and watch the Jet d'Eau, one of the tallest fountains in the world."

Aceline looks at the fountain. "Wow, you sure know your Lake Geneva facts! How high up does the water shoot up from the Jet d'Eau?"

"Almost 100 m. While this side of the lake is nice and you can see some of the Alpine mountains, the scenery on the eastern side is breathtaking. The eastern end has higher and bolder mountains, including the snowy peaks of Mont Blanc that are not visible on the lake's western side. Tomorrow we can take the train and go sightseeing on the eastern shore of Lake Geneva."

"I look forward to that. What are all these pictures on stands along the lake's walkway?"

"At various times, the WHO and other organizations involved in Global Health display pictures taken throughout the globe by their staff and others. We can go look at them before we head over to the Gardens."

For the next half-hour, they look at enlarged photos highlighting how people live in some of the poorest countries in the world. Aceline finds these pictures emotionally moving. "The picture of an elderly Ethiopian woman carrying a bundle of sticks on her back reminds me of the time I spent in Ethiopia years ago. The country used to be very green with many forests. Now, most of the trees are gone and the land is barren. This, and the severe poverty, breaks my heart."

"I know, but I am hopeful Ethiopia will do better going forward. The country is leading the way in Africa by creating a functional universal healthcare system."

"How are they doing that?"

"They developed a system where they select people in various communities and give them medical training over ten months in various facets of basic healthcare. After their training is complete, they provide preventive care, including vaccination, nutritional advice, and other basic items, to a group of families. These community trainees also have access to other healthcare workers with more training when needed."

"I should think about how to implement that in the DRC. How well has that worked?"

"The program has been successful in many, but not all, Ethiopian communities. It is being further refined."

David and Aceline finish looking at the pictures and then cut across the grounds of the Parc Barton on the left to the Conservatoire et Jardin Botanique. They enter the park at the corner of Rue de Lausanne and Avenue de la Paix. "Would you like to explore the garden before getting something to eat?"

"Is there time to see the entire garden today?"

"No, but we can see part of it today and come back another day."

"Lead on."

"Sometimes after I finish work, I walk down to the Botanical Gardens to find some tranquility. The Gardens has been at this site since the early 1900s and its 69 acres are home to thousands of different species of plants and trees that bloom at different times throughout the year. Sections of the Botanical Garden include the Animal Park, Arboretum, Garden of Smell and Touch, the Herbarium that includes medicinal plants, Rose Garden, and many more. We can see a few of these areas today and I prefer if you chose."

"Let's go to the Garden of Smell and Touch and then the medicinal plant section."

They walk into the first area, touching and gathering in the various scents from the plants. David notices Aceline has a continuous smile on her face and is hesitant to suggest they move on. After 45 minutes, Aceline tells David she is ready to go to the medicinal plant area. Once there, David mentions the Botanical Conservatory has a special interest in medicinal plants from Paraguay.

"Do you know why?"

"It has been a few years since I read about it, but my understanding is Emil Hassler was a Swiss physician who became interested in the flora of Paraguay. He visited the country on many occasions starting in the late 1800s and developed a collection containing almost all of Paraguay's plant species. After his death in 1937, the botanical collection was donated to this botanic garden. Paraguay's indigenous population used many of these plants for medicinal purposes."

"David, I am impressed with your knowledge. If your new position at the WHO doesn't pan out, I think you would make a lovely tour guide."

David laughs and asks Aceline if she would like to eat lunch at the Garden café. They walk over to the café and sit at one of the outside tables where a waiter takes their order. Aceline decides this is a good time to talk about wedding plans. "Every time I talk with my parents, their first question is whether we have set a date for our wedding."

"Do you have a date in mind?"

"What do you think about Saturday, December 23?"

"I can make it work. Do you want to get married in France?"

"That would be great. Can you take a week off after we get married for our honeymoon?"

"Can do. Do you have a place in mind?"

"I loved our short time in the Alps this past December, but wherever you want would be fine."

"The Alps, it is."

"I've been thinking about talking with my boss at Médecins Sans Frontières (MSF) about taking a leave of absence starting at the beginning of December."

"Do you know how long you want to take off?"

"I'm not sure. I realize in your new position you travel a lot, but still spend the majority of your time in Geneva. I think it would be great if we can both be together in the same city. I'm going to find out if there is a job with MSF based out of Geneva. If not, I might look for other global non-profit healthcare jobs based in Geneva."

"I think living in the same city would be great. I recognize you are making a sacrifice for me so if you don't find something you like in

Geneva, then I'll look for a job wherever you find something you like. One way or the other we will work this out so we are together."

Aceline and David finish lunch and start walking up to the WHO headquarters. Along the way, they pass the UN Geneva Headquarters, the second-largest of the four major UN office headquarters around the globe. Across the street from the UN is the Place des Nations square. The granite slabs in various colors symbolize the diversity of nations. Multiple small water jets shoot water upwards and in the center of the square stands a very tall chair with three normal legs and a fourth leg that is missing its bottom half.

"David, what is the story behind this chair?"

"The chair is a symbol for the campaign against landmines."

"Wow. The chair sends a powerful message. I cared for too many children and adults who lost one or both legs after stepping on a landmine. These landmines were put in the ground during past conflicts. Most have been removed, but some remain."

They continue walking as they turn onto Avenue Appia. David points out the International Red Cross Headquarters and Red Crescent Museum. He notes that part of the museum details the Red Cross's role in providing care for trauma victims affected by emergencies caused by wars, weather and other disasters.

Aceline shares an idea with David. "The Red Cross might be an alternative place for me to look for a job if things don't work out with MSF. I know there is not enough time to go today, but I would still like to spend some time in the museum to learn more about the work the Red Cross does."

"Always thinking ahead. We can come back later this week."

Aceline looks at David. "Actually, I'm always thinking of us."

David hugs her and they continue walking up the hill for ten minutes and then turn right onto the driveway leading to the WHO's main entrance and office buildings.

Aceline is surprised at what she sees. "I had a different picture of what it would look like. The main entrance has a lot of glass, but most of the other buildings have a concrete bunker look. How old is the WHO?"

"The WHO was established in 1948 and housed at the UN Headquarters, which we walked by a few minutes ago. Eventually, it became clear that the WHO had outgrown its accommodations, and the World Health Assembly passed a resolution to initiate the construction of a new headquarters building. Jean Tschumi, a Swiss architect, won the competition to design the headquarters. He drew up the plans but died before the construction was finished in 1966. The building of some additional annexes has occurred since then. I will give you a tour of the main building and then we can go underground to my office in the L annex."

They enter the main entrance and David takes out his identification badge. He takes Aceline by the security area so she can get a visitors' badge. The main floor is enclosed by glass walls and outside there is a patio. Tables inside and outside the building are occupied by groups of people, most of who appear to be doing work in small groups. Across from these tables is a café and above it is a veranda where most of the people are sitting individually. As they pass a set of elevators, David notes that the office of the Director-General is on the seventh floor of this building. David takes Aceline to the WHO library at the end of the main floor hallway where people are working on computers. After they leave the library, they turn right and go down a flight of stairs into the main WHO meeting room. There is a large circular table in the middle of the room and then rows of seating surrounding the circular table.

"Is this where the World Health Assembly meets?"

"This room is actually not big enough to be the venue for the World Health Assembly since there are 194 countries and several times the number of people who attend the meeting. That meeting takes place in a bigger room at the UN Geneva campus. However, the World Health Assembly Executive Board, composed of 35 members chosen by the entire assembly, meet in this room."

"What does the World Health Assembly and the Executive Board do?"

"The Assembly is responsible for approving major health policies proposed by the Director-General. Additionally, the World Health Assembly determines who will serve as Director-General, a five-year position that is renewable only once."

"What else is the room used for?"

"The WHO frequently requires consultation from outside experts on various topics related to global health. One example I am familiar with is: after the 2009 pandemic, the Director-General decided there was a need for a new pandemic influenza plan to improve the ability of all countries to deal with the next pandemic. In 2011, the World Health Assembly adopted the Pandemic Influenza Preparedness Framework. Over the next five years, the WHO staff and consultants used this framework to guide the development of recommendations aimed at increasing the ability of countries to detect potential new pandemic strains of influenza virus and to gain access to vaccines, drugs and other life-saving products. This effort included three meetings in this room to deal with the problems identified during the development of the plan. Similar consultations in other areas of health, including nutrition, global warming, and maternal health, occur in this room."

David and Aceline leave this meeting room and head over to his office through a tunnel system connecting the various annex office buildings. They pass by a storage area containing office supplies, and make several turns before they take an elevator up to his office on the first floor. Aceline follows David into the office and he asks her if she wants to sit in one of the chairs next to his desk. However, she keeps looking out the office window and then at the desk and table in his office.

"David, is that the main building across the street?"

"Yes."

"It seems very close given how long it took us to get through the tunnels to get here."

"If we walked outside instead of through the tunnel, we could have taken a more direct line."

"Papers, folders and books are all over your office."

"Are you surprised my office looks chaotic?"

"Your apartment is tidy but this office is a mess."

David finds her comment amusing. "You are witness to the anarchy of working in the area of global emergencies. There is actually a method to my madness, but I admit, everyone else, including my administrative assistant, has trouble finding things in this office. When I leave work and go home, I need the serenity of an uncluttered space."

"You are a fascinating man. So Tour Guide David, what's the history of the WHO's involvement in global health?"

"The WHO is a specialized agency that is the part of the UN system specifically focused on global public health. Prior to the creation of the WHO, its predecessor, the Health Organization, was an agency of the League of Nations. The current version of the WHO, with its headquarters in Geneva, began in 1948. The WHO's mandate over health issues is very broad and includes mitigating the effects of communicable and non-communicable diseases. Now, we come to where you choose your own adventure part of this tour. Which of those two do you want to hear about first?"

"Communicable diseases."

"My personal favorite. The WHO has a leading role in controlling and eliminating communicable diseases. The eradication of smallpox in 1980 is the most impressive achievement, but other work includes promoting the use of prevention and treatment methods to decrease various infectious diseases, including tuberculosis, malaria, polio, and onchocerciasis — the parasitic worm that causes blindness, measles and HIV.

"For my own division, the WHO's primary objective in natural and man-made emergencies is to coordinate with member states and other stakeholders to reduce avoidable loss of life and the burden of disease and disability. Working with national governments, and with the help of donor organizations, we try to improve governance, financing, staffing, and management during emergencies. We do this based on the evidence that is available to guide emergency policies. We also strive to ensure improved access, quality and use of medical products and technologies."

"That sounds like quite the important mission. What about non-communicable diseases?"

"That involves multiple areas, including sexual and reproductive health, development and aging, nutrition, food security, occupational health, environmental health, substance abuse, and trauma prevention and care."

"How many people work for the WHO?"

"The WHO employs approximately 8,500 people in 147 countries to carry out its mission in the six different regions. Most of these people are in low-income countries. There usually is one WHO country office in the capital, occasionally accompanied by satellite-offices in the provinces or sub-regions of the country. The country office consists of one WHO representative and several health experts, both foreign and local, as well as the necessary support staff. The main functions of WHO country offices include being the primary adviser to that country's government in matters of health and pharmaceutical policies."

"I had no idea how big the WHO was. How is all of that financed?"

"The WHO's budget last year was around $4 billion, of which approximately 25% comes from member states with the United States, Japan, Germany, United Kingdom and France contributing the largest amounts. The rest of the budget comes from private donors such as the Gates Foundation. The problem with this type of donation is that the donor usually directs the money to specific projects. This decreases the flexibility of the Director-General to redirect money when unexpected events occur. This is particularly problematic for my group, given the increasing numbers of global emergencies. I frequently need to request additional monies that are not in the budget and the leadership of the WHO spends a lot of time trying to raise these additional funds."

"That seems really constraining. Aren't there contingency funds within the budget to deal with these emergencies?"

"Yes, but for the past two decades, the increasing number of emergencies means there are never enough funds. We can talk more about this at dinner, but right now I would like you to meet some of the people I work with."

"Sounds great!"

For the rest of the afternoon, David takes Aceline to various offices on the same floor where she meets many of his colleagues in the Emergency Planning division. They begin walking home at 6 p.m. and along the way, they stop for dinner at Aux 5 Sens, an African restaurant near Gare Cornavin, the main train station.

"This is one of my favorite restaurants in Geneva. Their lamb chop dish is superb."

"I'm starving and lamb sounds yummy. You order the meal and I will pick the wine."

The server takes their order and Aceline grabs David's hand. "This has been a great day. I've learned so much about Geneva and the WHO. I also loved getting to meet some of the people you talked about when we were in the DRC. They're very dedicated and are obviously fond of you."

"When we were in Philippe's office and you went to the bathroom, he told me you were an incredible catch, and I better marry you before someone else does."

"Have you told everyone in your division we're getting married?"

"Philippe is one of my best friends and I told him soon after I proposed to you. I didn't ask him to keep it quiet so I'm certain most people know. He does enjoy a bit of gossip," David says as he winks at Aceline.

"It's been a long time since I've felt this good. After dinner, we should head back to the apartment so I can show you just how happy I am."

David and Aceline spend the rest of the week exploring various places in Geneva and nearby towns. Aceline also starts looking into job opportunities at the MSF and Red Cross headquarters in Geneva. The day she leaves to go back to the DRC, the mood is a little somber since neither of them has any vacation days until the second half of the year. They make temporary plans for their next time together and decide the only way to deal with their separation is to talk every day by phone until then.

Chapter 11

Geneva, Switzerland, Summer of 2017

The World Health Assembly Director-General Selection subcommittee worked for over a year to develop a list of Director-General candidates to present for consideration to all the countries that make up the World Health Assembly. During the annual World Health Assembly meeting in May 2017, the members chose Dr. Negasi Kebede, as the new Director-General, from a list of six final candidates. He officially assumes the position on July 1, 2017.

Dr. Kebede has been working on his new five-year plan to improve global health since his appointment. David finally gets to meet with him in mid-August. Upon entering his office, David introduces himself and then adds, "I have heard many good things about your prior work in the areas of public health and universal health programs. I'm delighted to have the chance to work with you. I hope you had a chance to read the summary I sent you on the current status of ongoing emergencies and our updated Human Emergencies Strategy Plan."

"David, I heard you are doing a really nice job in your new position. I did read your summary of the updated plan and think it will help us be better able to proactively, rather than reactively, deal with the increasing number of outbreaks. During my interviews with the World Health Assembly Selection subcommittee, I emphasized the urgency of improving the response to these outbreaks. The part of your plan that includes social scientists to improve our ability to interact with different communities is excellent and I intend to create an internal group within the WHO with expertise in communications and implementation of programs. This group will not only help with outbreaks, but also fits in nicely with our goal to expand universal healthcare to another one billion people globally."

"Do you think funding the plan will be a problem?"

"The WHO has received inadequate funding for many years and increasing our current funding is key to many parts of my five-year plan. This is particularly true for its role in overseeing the response to various emergencies. I emphasized to the World Health Assembly and our various donors the need to halt the deterioration of the core funding provided by all the countries so that we can become less dependent on the voluntary contributions of outside donors designated to specific programs or problems. The current budget constraints are resulting in insufficient flexibility to deal with new emergencies or other unforeseen problems that arise. The five-year plan I am working on will contain a transparent budget indicating the money needed, including contingency funding, and how it will be spent."

"Please let me know if there is anything I can do to help."

"Next month, I will be going to New York for the annual UN General Assembly session. I will meet with the UN Secretary-General before the General assembly session begins. He wants to talk about the status of the WHO Pandemic Influenza Plan. Can you give me a brief background summary of the WHO's Pandemic Influenza Plan and where things currently stand?"

"Sure. In 2006, the WHO started to address the lack of influenza vaccines available for low-income countries during an influenza pandemic. The creation of the Global Action Plan for Influenza Vaccines was a ten-year initiative to help deal with this issue. Development of the plan occurred in collaboration with outside experts on influenza and public health, as well as vaccine manufacturers and funding agencies. The 2009 influenza pandemic highlighted many of the problems that the original plan did not alleviate, including the scarcity of vaccines available for use in low-income countries. This past winter, the Third WHO Consultation of the Global Action Plan for Influenza Vaccines meeting took place in Geneva to determine what progress has occurred since the 2009 pandemic. During the past decade, the global capacity to produce influenza vaccines increased from 1.5 billion doses to more than 6 billion doses, and the WHO has reached an agreement with some of the vaccine manufacturers to set aside a portion of the vaccine for low-income countries. Additionally, the number of countries with pandemic plans increased from 74 to 115, but only one low-income country has finished their pandemic plan."

"Has this information been presented to the World Health Assembly recently?"

"The information was presented at the annual meeting this year. The Assembly members appreciated the progress made to date, but remained very concerned that a great deal of work is still required. They noted that vaccine production falls short of the Global Action Plan goal to immunize 70% of the world's population with two doses of vaccine that are anticipated to be required to produce an effective immune response. They requested further work be done to reduce barriers to vaccine access and affordability and to further increase vaccine production capacity. The Assembly members also highlighted the need for the development of a more effective vaccine. A recent survey of the members asked what global issues were of greatest concern. Pandemic influenza preparedness was ranked in the top 10."

The Director-General is surprised. "Given that the 2009 influenza pandemic was not severe and all the other problems that cause substantial mortality on an annual basis, I would not have thought this would be in the top 10 list of concerns of the countries."

"The 1918 influenza pandemic impact on the world was enormous because of the very high number of deaths and disruption of the global economy. The 1918 pandemic caused 40–100 million deaths globally. The highest death rate was in young adults."

"Was this true for wealthy as well as poor countries?"

"Yes. Our most reliable data is from high-income countries. For example, in the US, approximately 500,000 people died and the average age of death was 28 years of age. This resulted in a decrease in life expectancy of 12 years."

"Did similar decreases in life expectancy occur in subsequent influenza pandemics?"

"The last three pandemics in 1957, 1968 and 2009 were less severe and only the 2009 pandemic had a predilection for deaths in young adults. However, even these less severe pandemics caused millions of deaths globally."

The Director-General takes a minute to consider what he has learned. "That makes sense. I can see why countries list influenza pandemics as one of their top concerns."

"Indeed, and it's not only the number of deaths that worry the countries. The impact of the 1918 pandemic on the global economy was severe and given the marked increase in economic globalization, there is currently a high level of concern a worldwide pandemic will devastate the economies of all countries."

"Has our ability to impact the severity of a future pandemic improved?"

David knows there has been some progress, but much remains to be done. "That's a mixed bag. There are many problematic issues remaining. The next pandemic, if severe, could infect billions of people and overwhelm the capacity of the healthcare system in each country to provide the needed care. Sufficient quantities of a vaccine for worldwide use against the specific strain of influenza virus causing the pandemic would likely take at least a year to produce. The quantity of antiviral medicine needed for those who become ill remains inadequate. With so many people becoming ill, the stress on the workforce needed to maintain critical infrastructure and services would be tremendous. All countries will be affected, but low-income counties will be impacted the most."

The Director-General thinks out loud. "We need billions of dollars to deal with influenza and other types of emergencies. My biggest concern is that some of the major donor high-income countries are promoting a return to nationalism and turning their focus internally. This may well result in decreasing their support for global issues, including health. I plan to discuss this issue with the UN Secretary-General. He is someone I have known for years and whom I think can help us determine the best approach to raising the necessary funds. I would like you to come to the

UN with me and attend part of my meeting with the Secretary-General. Your knowledge about pandemic planning will help answer questions the Secretary-General may have."

David hadn't anticipated this request. "When will the meeting occur?"

"The last week in September. Can you make it?"

"I'll make any needed adjustments to my calendar."

"David, does the Pandemic Influenza Plan need further work before we travel to the UN?"

"My group is working on it now and I'll make sure it is finished before we go to New York."

***

David calls Aceline that evening. He tells her about his conversation with the new Director-General earlier in the day. He realizes they had planned to spend a week in September together in Paris and asks if she would be okay changing the venue to New York. She likes the idea and they agree to meet there. David realizes how much he likes their nightly calls, but as soon as they are finished, all he can think about is how much he misses her. Waiting until September is going to be hard. He hopes burying himself in work will make the time go by faster.

During the next six weeks, David works with Philippe and two other members of his team who are influenza experts on refining the WHO's Pandemic Influenza Plan. David has talked with Richard Huff on multiple occasions during this time to get his ideas and feedback on the plan. A few days before his New York trip, David sends the revised plan to the Director-General via email. He includes an Executive Summary of the changes made compared to the previous Pandemic Influenza Plan and asks if he wants him to make a presentation to the Secretary-General. The Director-General indicates that rather than a formal presentation, he just wants David to be ready to give a brief overview of the Pandemic Influenza Plan and answer any questions the Secretary-General asks.

Chapter 12

New York City US, September 2017

The Director-General and David fly from Geneva to Newark Airport in New Jersey the day before their meeting with Martim Barcellos, the UN Secretary-General. They grab a taxi to the Millennium Hilton hotel located a few blocks from the UN headquarters where the Director-General is staying. David has booked a hotel several miles away since the General Assembly meeting will be ongoing when Aceline arrives in two days, and driving near the UN will become impossible due to security blockades. The Director-General asks David to meet him in the main lobby of the UN tomorrow, 15 minutes prior to the scheduled meeting with the Secretary-General.

The taxi cab driver takes David to the Paramount Hotel near Broadway. He chose this hotel since it was near the theater district and he has purchased tickets to a Broadway play. Once he gets into his hotel room, he takes a shower and then considers going out to get dinner. However, it is approaching 7 p.m. in New York, which is 1 a.m. in Geneva, and he is tired. He orders room service and then falls asleep soon after eating.

The following morning his phone alarm wakes him from a deep sleep at 7:30 a.m. He gets dressed and then has breakfast in the hotel. He leaves the hotel before 9 a.m. to be certain he has time to walk over to the UN and meet the Director-General for their meeting with the Secretary-General. When he is within ten blocks of the UN, he notes all the roads have barricades and are teeming with police. Only cars with diplomatic plates can get closer to the UN and many people are getting out of taxis and walking along with him to the UN plaza.

He arrives at the UN a few minutes early and sees that the Director-General is already in the atrium. They take an elevator up to the Secretary-General's office and the receptionist leads them into a conference room. A few minutes later, the Secretary-General joins them and warmly greets the Director-General. "Negasi, my friend. It's been a long time since we have been in the same room together."

They embrace each other. "Indeed, Martim, too long."

The Director-General then introduces David to the Secretary-General, who is aware David will be joining them for the first part of the meeting. "David, thank you for taking the time to come to New York. I am interested to hear your thoughts about what we can do to help all countries deal with pandemic influenza."

"It is an honor to meet you and I appreciate you inviting me to this meeting. The Director-General asked me to give you a brief overview of pandemic influenza and then answer any questions you have. Unlike most of the outbreaks we deal with that are limited in their geographical spread, influenza pandemics rapidly spread throughout the world. Depending on their severity, they can result in very high numbers of deaths and widespread social and economic disruption."

The Secretary-General doesn't wait for David to finish his overview. "David, I know the influenza virus caused the worst pandemic in recorded history just about a century ago. What was the mortality rate in this pandemic and how does it compare to epidemic influenza?"

"The estimated mortality rate for the 1918 pandemic was 2.5% as compared to the lower ~0.1% mortality we see in most years due to seasonal influenza. The population of the world in 1918 was around 1.8 billion compared to more than 7.5 billion now. If the next influenza pandemic causes a mortality rate anywhere close to 2.5%, there could be many millions of deaths globally despite the fact we now have drugs to treat influenza early on in the pandemic and the availability of a vaccine probably within the first year to decrease the impact of the disease. The greatest impact will be in low- and middle-income countries."

"Given that high-income countries are affected by influenza pandemics, how much does the planning process of these countries help low- and middle-income countries?"

"Their planning helps and hurts other countries. Their investments help develop tests, drugs and vaccines for use in a pandemic. However, the most recent influenza pandemic in 2009 highlighted some of the major inequities between high-income and other countries. The wealthy countries and some middle-income countries have contracts with vaccine companies to buy vaccines as soon as they come off the manufacturing lines. The production of a vaccine can only begin once we know the exact strain of influenza causing the pandemic and it takes four to six months to produce the vaccine. During the 2009 pandemic, the WHO created an agreement with vaccine manufacturers to obtain 10% of the vaccine as it comes off the manufacturing production lines. Since more than 80% of the world's population live in low- or middle-income countries, only a small percentage of them received the vaccine. This inequity issue also applies to drugs, healthcare supplies, including ventilators, and other items needed to deal with an influenza pandemic."

"What has been done since then to improve this situation?"

"Currently, the high-income countries in North America and Europe are all creating individual plans for their own country, but there is little coordination between these countries. The situation is even worse in developing countries where over 75 countries have yet to create a pandemic plan. The WHO has organized several meetings where leading international experts are working with us on the best way for the global community to address strengthening influenza pandemic preparedness in all countries. There has been discussion about developing new types of influenza vaccines that would take less time to manufacture and be available in large enough quantities to vaccinate the entire global population. The development of this type of vaccine will take at least a decade and a large amount of new funding. My concern about this has been further heightened by the recent trend of some high-income countries to focus internally only on its own population and decrease the money they donate for global causes."

"Negasi told me you are working on a five-year plan to more effectively intervene in all types of outbreaks. Can you give me a brief summary of any parts of the plan that could impact influenza pandemics in low-income countries?"

"Absolutely. Several of our recommendations could help in an influenza pandemic. One recommendation involves technologies and one, in particular, could have a marked impact on influenza pandemics.

"Tell me more about this one."

"The current influenza vaccines must be kept at 2°C to 8°C. Exposure to temperatures outside this range results in decreased vaccine potency. Therefore, transportation of influenza vaccines to clinics requires refrigerated vehicles, and then they must be stored at the clinic at this temperature until they are administered intramuscularly to recipients. During a pandemic, many people receive the vaccine each day and this increases the risk of disease transmission between those coming to the clinic. A new technology involving the use of microarray patches would allow us to give the vaccines intradermally, rather than intramuscularly."

"What advantages do the microarray patches offer over the current way we administer the influenza vaccine?"

"The patches have the potential to revolutionize the way we give influenza and many other vaccines. The microarray patches are easy to apply to the skin. This makes giving the vaccine easier for healthcare workers. Additionally, the needles on the patches are very small and barely penetrate the skin. Unlike the longer needles used for intramuscular injection, less than 10% of people experience any pain when microarray patches are applied. Some parents who bring their infant to a clinic for the first time don't come back because they don't like the way vaccine injections make their child cry. These patches will also help increase the vaccination rate in children and adults who have needle phobias."

"Are there other advantages of microarray patches that could help in a flu pandemic?"

"The influenza vaccine contains two antigens, the hemagglutinin and neuraminidase proteins used to generate the immune response. The developers of the microarray patches have come up with a method to freeze-dry these proteins onto the patches and this allows them to be heat stable at up to 40°C for at least two weeks. This eliminates the need for refrigerated transport and storage of the vaccine. These patches take up much less space than vaccine vials and, therefore, the number of vaccine doses one can carry in transport vehicles is substantially greater. During a pandemic, these patches could be also sent through the mail service. In places without mail service, the patches could be taken into the village by someone who can also demonstrate how to apply the patch."

"Are microarray patches being developed for other vaccines?"

"Yes. Work is currently underway to develop microarray patches for measles-rubella, rabies and human papilloma virus vaccines. Potentially other vaccines we now give by injection could also be put on a microarray patch."

"How does the immune response of vaccines on microarray patches compare to other routes for the injection of vaccines?"

"The studies done so far have suggested that the immunologic response is equal or better when given intradermally."

"This sounds really promising. It seems to me that the microarray patches could be transformational, not only for dealing with pandemics, but also routine immunization. How long will it take to bring these microarray patch vaccines to market?"

"To date, the microarray vaccine studies have only been done in animals. There is a planned study using the influenza vaccine in a Phase 1 human trial and we need more of these studies with influenza and other vaccines. All of this will require a major cooperative effort involving global health funders, scientists, regulators and the industry. Without this cooperation and a large amount of new funding, this will take decades."

"I am impressed by the tremendous potential these microarray patches have for improving the vaccine program for pandemic influenza and also many other vaccine-preventable diseases. What can I do to help move this along?"

David decides to express the severe stress the decreased WHO funding has already had on his group. "I need to put several people onto the microarray patch project, but the budget cuts have forced the WHO to freeze the hiring of new people. For my division, this has also impeded our ability to respond to the marked increase in emergencies. Recently, one of the best people in the division told me he was suffering from burnout and requested time off for the rest of the year. Another person in my group told me she was looking for other jobs because the increasingly heavy workload was affecting not only her, but also her family."

"David, I hear the exasperation in your voice and this feeling is increasingly being expressed by others working in different divisions in the UN. I'm very concerned that the funding for global health from some of the high-income countries is decreasing. One of the major points of my upcoming speech before the General Assembly relates to the impact decreased funding is having on the most important problems facing the world, including global warming and health. I am going to highlight the increasing number of global emergencies and the lack of adequate funding in our budget to deal with these problems. My predecessor told me that most leaders of high-income countries understand dealing with these regional outbreaks is important, both from an ethical and economic impact basis. However, in the last few years, the leadership of some of these countries has changed and they are decreasing their support of global crisis unless it directly affects their country."

The Director-General then adds, "The US President recently announced he is considering a 25% decrease in foreign aid. The US has been engaged in international health activities for more than a century and is today the largest funder of global health programs worldwide. This past year, the US budget for global health was over $10 billion. However, it actually decreased this year. How can we convince him this is a terrible idea?"

The Secretary-General immediately responds, "I have given this considerable thought. Currently, almost two billion people live where there are protracted crises, such as infectious disease outbreaks, droughts causing severe famine, and armed conflicts. Many of these high-income countries, including the US, are now experiencing large numbers of desperate people trying to immigrate into their countries. In my talk to the General Assembly and in separate meetings with the leaders of these high-income countries, I will forcibly make the case that investing in low-income countries is not only the right thing to do, but will help decrease the number of people trying to migrate to their countries."

The Director-General notes how he may be able to help, "I have a meeting with the US Secretary of State while I am in New York and hope to make many of the same points you just expressed. I think my best argument is that reducing funding for international programs would have far-reaching effects that ultimately impede the international and domestic policy agendas of the US. These programs encompass many activities in addition to foreign aid and are key to establishing and maintaining positive relations with other countries. These relationships contribute to increased economic opportunities in the US, better international cooperation, and thereby enhances national security."

"Nagasi, I hope that between the two of us we can drive home these points. In the meantime, I will try to get the US President to meet with me individually this week while he is in New York. I think I will use David's example of what the next pandemic, whether due to influenza or some other organism, could do to all countries if we don't invest in pandemic planning."

The Secretary-General looks at David. "I greatly appreciate the update on what your group is doing regarding infectious disease emergencies. I need to continue the meeting with the Director-General to discuss other issues. However, I think you should consider extending the current five-year plan to a comprehensive ten-year plan. Doing this will ensure there is a plan in place for the next Secretary-General and Director-General when our terms expire. In the meantime, the Director-General and I will do everything we can to raise the necessary funds so there is enough money in the annual budgets to implement your plan and that there is no need to go begging every time a new crisis occurs."

David leaves the UN building and starts walking back to his hotel. He thinks the meeting went well, but sends an email to the Director-General to get some feedback. His thoughts quickly switch to Aceline, who will be arriving this afternoon. He knows she has been to New York City before, but other than going to a Broadway play, he realizes that he has once again neglected to ask her what she would like to do. He decides to surprise her by meeting her at Newark airport rather than waiting for her at the hotel. He uses Google Map to determine if he has enough time to take a train from Penn Station to the Newark airport if he does not stop first at the hotel. He arrives at the airport just a few minutes before her plane arrives and goes to the luggage area. When Aceline comes out of the Customs into the luggage area, she does not see David. He quietly comes up behind her.

"Lady, do I know you?"

Aceline turns around, breaks out in a huge smile, and hugs him. "I thought I was meeting you at the hotel."

"The meeting with the UN Secretary-General finished on time and I decided I could either wait at the hotel or take the train to the airport and spend some more time with you."

"Good choice. How did the meeting go?"

"While I was waiting for you to come through US Customs, I got an email from the Director-General who said that my participation at the meeting was very helpful. Now, I want you to promise me that for the rest of our week together in New York, we will not discuss work."

"Perfect."

"Once we get your luggage, we can take a taxi back to the hotel so you can take a nap. After that we can go to dinner and discuss what places you would like to visit while we are here."

The ride to the hotel takes more than 90 minutes due to heavy traffic going from New Jersey to New York through the Lincoln tunnel. As they cross into Manhattan and approach 7th Avenue, Aceline notices it takes about five minutes for the taxi to move a block. "My friend who lives in Manhattan told me at times the traffic is so bad that the cars don't move. I think the term she used was gridlock."

"We are actually near the Broadway theater district where we are going tomorrow night to see the play, *Hamilton*, I told you about on the phone. This area is often very congested and at times, even the pedestrians are walking so slowly they appear to be in gridlock. Eventually, everything does move, but we need to account for the traffic if we want to be somewhere at a specific time. For many of the places we might visit this week, we can either walk or take the subway."

"No problem. I packed walking shoes."

They finally arrive at the hotel and go up to the room. Aceline notices that the room is bigger than the typical European hotel room, but is otherwise not much different. She quickly unpacks as David sits in the only chair watching her. She starts to undress and looks right at him. "Are you going to let me shower alone?"

David cracks a big smile. "Not a chance."

After the shower, they lie down in the bed and quickly fall asleep. They wake up just after 8 p.m. and put on some casual clothes to go to dinner. David asks the concierge to recommend a laid-back place for dinner that is close by. He recommends Ellen's Stardust Diner for its 1950s themed atmosphere, including singing waiters and a wide variety of American dishes.

They walk a few blocks and look at the menu posted on the outside window. The menu includes breakfast options served all day, which Aceline finds particularly appealing. Once seated, she orders the Brooklyn Pride with scrambled eggs and American cheese on a bagel. David gets the North Carolina Tarheel sandwich made of barbeque pulled pork with coleslaw. David suggests they both get an Old Fashion New York Egg Cream to drink. While waiting for their meal, they enjoy the lively atmosphere of the restaurant, including the waiters singing a variety of songs. The waiter brings their meals and they ask him about the singing. He tells them many of the people working at the restaurant are aspiring actors. They enjoy their job because they get to practice their craft while working and the tips tend to be very good. Dinner is great, but as the clock approaches 10 p.m., they decide to ask their waiter for a check and then go back to the hotel. "How big a tip should I leave?"

"Good question. Until our waiter mentioned tips, I forgot that people leave tips in America."

"Yip. Unlike Europe, waiters here depend on tips to survive."

"Our waiter was excellent. How much do people usually leave for a tip?"

"I think 15% to 25%."

"What do you think about 30%?"

"My fiancé is a generous woman. Just another one of your traits I love."

David pays for dinner and they start to walk back to the hotel. "What places do you want to visit while in New York?"

"I was ten years old the only other time I was here and it was with my parents. I remember taking a boat to see the Statue of Liberty, going to a huge toy store, and going to a couple of Broadway shows, but not much else."

"Do you remember walking through Central Park?"

"Not really and I would definitely like to do that. On the plane ride over here, I read about things to do, and the Museum of Modern Art and the High Line in Chelsea were high on my list. Have you been to any of these places before?"

"All my previous visits to New York were for business. I do know several good restaurants, but other than Central Park, I have not been to the places you mentioned."

"We can skip Central Park if you want."

"Actually, Central Park was on my list. It's a very large park with lots of people that make being there interesting. We can go there tomorrow."

"What else is on your list?"

"Besides seeing *Hamilton* on Broadway tomorrow night, I would like to go to the 9/11 Memorial Museum and also watch the New York Giants play American football."

"Have you ever been to an American football game?"

"When I was in New York the last time, a colleague invited me to come to a Sunday afternoon football party at his apartment. There were about four couples at the party sitting watching the game. They were nice enough to explain the rules of the game to me between their yelling and screaming for and at their team. Since then I watched some games on television and actually quite like the game. Would you be willing to go if I can get tickets?"

"I am always up for trying something new."

"You said one of your friends lives in New York. Should we invite her to one of these places or to go out to eat?

"I spoke with her last week about places we might want to visit and asked her to come to dinner with us. Unfortunately, she is out of town this week. Do you want to meet up with the person who invited you to the football party?"

"I saw him last week while he was at a meeting at the WHO. He is in China this week."

"We can invite both of our friends and their spouses to our wedding if you want."

"Great idea. We are almost at our hotel. Do you want to go up to the room or do something else?"

"I think we need to get to sleep so that we can get up early and explore Central Park."

***

The following morning, David and Aceline eat breakfast at the hotel and then walk north along 7th Avenue to 59th Street where Central Park begins.

"David, before you woke up this morning, I read about Central Park. In the past few years, the city stopped allowing cars in the park, but you can ride bikes through three different loops. This would allow us to see much more of the Park."

"That should be fun. Where can we rent bikes?"

"There are lots of places including one at Columbus Circle, which is only a few blocks from here."

They rent the bikes from a Citibike station and enter the Park at Columbus Circle. They quickly reach the Full Loop, which is the longest of the three loops and runs for six miles. They ride through some shaded areas and notice there are multiple fields with people playing soccer and softball. They come to an area that includes the Central Park Carousel and Sailboat Pond. They get off their bikes to walk around. The park is full of people walking, riding bikes and sitting on benches or grass areas.

"Would you mind if we take a rowboat out on the pond?"

"I was thinking the same thing."

David rows the boat out to the north side of the pond. Aceline moves over to be closer to him. "This is a wonderful place. You lose the sense of being in one of the largest cities in the world. Watching the children on the carousel smiling and interacting with other children and their parents was heartwarming. Have you ever thought about being a parent?"

"Occasionally, but until now there hasn't been anyone I want to have a child with. How about you?"

Aceline wraps her arms around David and looks into his eyes. "Many times during the past year. Do you think we would make good parents?"

"I am not sure. Our careers are so time demanding. On the other hand, I used to wonder if I should even get married since work dominates so much of my time. I realize now that when we are together, I spend less time thinking about work."

"I feel the same way. We can talk more about this later, but right now we should get back on our bikes and see more of the park."

They finish the full loop and then on the way to the shorter Reservoir Loop they stop to get a pretzel and drink from one of the many vendors on the trail. The trail circles around the Jacqueline Kennedy Onassis Reservoir. They spend a few hours riding and sitting on a bench, taking in the beautiful lakefront views and the skyscrapers on the horizon. In the late afternoon, they take one of the exits out of the Park and return the bikes. They stop at a nearby café with an outside patio and order a slice of pizza and a glass of red wine. The sun is beginning to set as they finish eating.

"Are you ready to go back to the hotel so we can take a nap before dinner?"

"There is one more thing I would like to do before we head back to the hotel."

He takes Aceline's hand and they walk across 59th Street to the Park entrance. He approaches one of the horse-drawn carriages and chats with the driver. He then helps Aceline into the carriage. For the next hour, they snuggle under a blanket while they ride around part of the southeastern part of the Park. When the ride finishes, they take a taxi back to the hotel. They decide to order dinner in their room and soon thereafter fall asleep.

***

The following morning, Aceline and David head out to the Wall Street area in Manhattan to visit the 9/11 Memorial Museum. The 9/11 Museum opened on September 11, 2011, exactly ten years after the terrorist attack occurred. The Museum documents the story of the Al Qaeda-lead terrorist attack where two hijacked planes crashed into the World

Trade Center Twin Towers in New York City, a third hit the Pentagon in Washington, DC, and the fourth crashed near Shanksville, Pennsylvania, after passengers on the plane disrupted the attempted attack. They spend hours in the museum learning about the terrorist attack, the background stories on some of the 2,977 people who died during the attack, and the impact this event had on the entire country. David notices tears in Aceline's eyes on several occasions and when they leave the museum, he puts his arm around her shoulder. Are you sorry we went to the museum?

"No. It did make me wonder why the stories about those who died during the 9/11 attack made me cry when I see so much misery every day in our work and don't cry?"

"Very sick people seek our help during outbreaks and it forces us to focus on trying to save lives. There is little time to think about anything else. I did get depressed early in my career but quickly developed ways to keep heartbreaking thoughts out of my mind. The most useful coping mechanism for me is to keep remembering I am doing everything possible to prevent deaths."

Aceline agrees and adds, "I also remind myself nature is causing the deaths. The difference in the case of 9/11 was that the tragedy was due to humans rather than nature."

"When I saw tears in your eyes, I wondered why my eyes were dry. Do you think our coping mechanisms harden our hearts to these tragedies?"

"We all deal with tragedies differently. What I do know is you are a warm and wonderful person."

"Thanks and I promise the rest of the week will be all about having fun."

That night they go to see the play *Hamilton* at Roger theater on Broadway. The play is a rap lyrical musical that tells a story about the history of America during the early years after winning independence from England. As a lover of all things history, David is captivated by the play and hopes that Aceline feels the same way. After the play, they stop by a bar and order two glasses of white wine.

David is beaming. "My friend told me that the play was good, but good does not even begin to describe it. Telling the story through rap music was brilliant and I am not someone who normally listens to rap."

"I agree. Often when someone raves about a movie or play, I go in with high expectations and end up being disappointed. Not this time. The play portrays Alexander Hamilton in a positive light. I wonder how true it is."

"I'm not sure. The play is based on a biography written by Ron Chernow in 2004."

"Let's stop at a bookstore while we are in Manhattan and get the book. I can read it on my flight home."

"My understanding is the book is over 800 pages. It will take a while to read."

"No problem, I love having a good book to read while I'm in Africa."

"I look forward to hearing your synopsis."

Aceline laughs. "Making me do all the work."

***

The next day they take a taxi down to the High Line, which is a public park built on an elevated rail structure running from Gansevoort Street to 34th Steet on Manhattan's West Side. Aceline's friend recommended going to the High Line and she read about the area the night before. They walk through the Chelsea market and onto the High Line walkway. "I thought this would be a fun place to walk and now I can be your tour guide! For most of the 20th century, this was a freight rail line that transported materials to the factories and warehouses of the industrial West Side. The use of the railway stopped in 1980, and in 1999, the neighborhood residents worked with the New York City Department of Parks & Recreation to preserve the elevated rail track we are walking on now. They transformed the area into a public park that combines nature, art and design."

"The view of the Hudson River is great. How long is the walkway?"

"About one and a half miles. We can walk it now and look at the plants, art and architecture along the way."

About halfway along the walkway, they sit down on one of the benches and David notes an unusual futuristic-looking building with rounded glass corners and steel bands. He points to the building. "Do you know anything about that building?"

"Zaha Hadid is a famous Iraqi-British architect who has designed many high-rise structures that can be found in some of the major cities throughout the world. She, along with others in her company, designed this 11-story building for luxury condominiums."

"The building is amazing. Has she designed any buildings in Geneva?"

"I am not aware of any in Geneva. She has designed buildings in other European cities, including my hometown of Paris and in cities in Asia and the Middle East. She also has designed other types of buildings, including museums, sports centers, and composites of buildings for a large area within a city. Some of these buildings won prestigious architecture awards."

"I can imagine — this one alone is so creative looking. Do you know how much it costs to buy a condominium in that building?"

"It depends on the size, but I did not see any costing less than $5 million and one cost $50 million."

"That might be even more costly than in Geneva."

"Speaking of expensive living in Geneva... When we get married, do you want to stay in your apartment or move somewhere else?"

"I hadn't really thought about it. What would you like to do?"

"I like the location of the apartment, but it is a bit small. If we have a child, we need more than one bedroom."

"That's a really good point. I've been giving your question about having a child a fair amount of thought since you first asked me about it when we were together in Geneva a few months ago. I think I want children, but I want to get answers to two questions I have."

"Are they questions I can help answer?"

"The first one needs a factual answer. I am 42 years of age and you are 35. What does that mean as far as the risk of us having a child with Down syndrome or some other genetic defect? I think before we make a final decision we should meet with an obstetrician and hear what they say."

"Fair enough. What is your other question?"

"Our jobs put both of us at increased risk of dying from an infection. What will happen to our child if one or both of us die before he or she is an adult."

"Another great question. Let's both think about this more and we can discuss it later."

Aceline lays her head on David's shoulder and they sit on the bench in silence for what seems like a long time. Eventually, they exit the walkway by walking down a set of stairs onto the street. On their walk back to the hotel, they stop at a bookstore where Aceline finds the Alexander Hamilton biography they had discussed the previous night. When they are a block away from the hotel, Aceline tells David she wants to stop at a nearby store and will meet him back at their room.

When she gets back to the hotel, they order in-room dining. After dinner, Aceline goes into the bathroom. David thinks she is going to shower, but a few minutes later Aceline comes out wearing the negligee she just purchased and smiles at David. "Would you care to join me in bed?"

***

The following day, they walk over to the Museum of Modern Art. They spend hours walking through the multiple exhibitions that are on each of the building's six floors. After that, they stop at a restaurant and order dinner. "David, the museum was really different than the ones I have been to in Paris. I hope you enjoyed it as much as I did."

"I did. We spent over three hours in there and the time just flew by. I can't believe we have only two more days in New York before we have to go back to work. Tonight is the football game, but we can skip it if there are other things you want to do."

"No way. I want to experience American football in person, so don't even think about not taking me to the game. The only other activity left on my list is to walk across the Brooklyn Bridge into Dumbo at sunset."

"We can definitely do both."

They take the bus to MetLife Stadium to see the New York Giants play the Dallas Cowboys. The bus pulls into the parking lot two hours before the game starts and Aceline is surprised at how many fans are already there. "It looks like everyone is eating a meal before they even go to the game."

"Americans call this tailgating. My friends tell me fans come 3–4 hours before a game with cooking grills and make an entire meal that usually consists of various types of meat and a variety of side dishes and drinks. Have you been to a football game in Europe where people go to pubs to eat and drink before the game?"

"Yes, and some of those people are tipsy before they even enter the stadium."

"I suspect the same thing happens here."

"Isn't American football a different game than le football in France?"

"What we call le football, Americans call soccer. American football is a very different game and there is a lot of physical contact between players. Let's go into the stadium and find our seats and I will tell you more about how American football is played."

They enter the stadium and their seats are on the second level around the 30-yard line. David explains to Aceline the basic rules of American football, including how a team scores points. Based on her questions, he wonders if she will find the game too violent. During the first 15 minutes of the game, he tries to explain more about what is going on. He is surprised at how quickly she catches on and realizes she is clearly following the action of the field. At the end of the first half, they go to the concession stand to get some food.

"What would you like to eat and drink?"

"I want the full football experience — a hot dog and a beer." David breaks out laughing and she punches him in the arm. "You had better order the same thing for yourself."

"You seem to be having fun."

"The game is nothing like le football. There are breaks between each play and you don't hear fans singing for their team. The physical nature of the game is also very different, but I find it interesting. I can't believe how hard the running back and receivers are hit by the defensive players. The fans cheer the loudest when one of the Giant defensive players clobbers a Dallas offensive player."

"You really are into the game."

"What's there not to like? The game is intense and the fan reactions add to the atmosphere."

They go back to their seats for the second half. The Giants win the game by kicking a field goal with 20 seconds left in the game. The fans go crazy, screaming and high-fiving people near them. Ten minutes later, they head out to the parking lot to take the bus back to Manhattan. "I was worried you might not like it, but clearly I was wrong."

"Of all the places we went this week, this was the most unique and fun thing we did."

"You didn't find the 9/11 museum was unique?"

"The 9/11 museum was unique, but not fun."

"Got it."

"I can't believe tomorrow is our last full day in New York. I really want to buy some clothes before we walk across the Brooklyn Bridge tomorrow evening. Is that okay?"

"Being anywhere with you is always okay."

The next day they walk to Bloomingdale's in midtown Manhattan. Aceline spends an hour looking for clothes and shoes. After that, they take a taxi downtown to the Mystique Boutique on Canal Street.

"David, thanks for being so patient and helping me shop."

"I enjoyed the fashion show. Although, I doubt my opinion on clothes is worth much. What made you pick those two clothing stores from all the others in Manhattan?"

"My friend who lives here told me where she shops for clothes and we have similar taste."

They get something to eat and then decide to go to see *Spettacolo*, a documentary movie that focuses on a Tuscan village where residents put on an elaborate play about their own lives. After the movie ends in the early evening, they take the subway to the High Street-Brooklyn Bridge stop. They follow the signage to the pedestrian stairway and walk up to the Brooklyn Bridge walkway. The sun is setting as they begin their 1.5-mile walk to the Brooklyn side.

"Your idea of doing this at sunset was a stroke of genius. The view of the city building with its lights along with the boats on the East River is spectacular."

For a few minutes, they walk in silence, taking in the scenery. A bike rider startles them by yelling at them to move to the right. David takes Aceline hand and moves closer to the bridge railing. Aceline decides it is a good time to talk about their future together. "I think this is the perfect setting to start talking about our future together."

"I'm all ears."

"Would you be okay with a small wedding in the backyard of my parents' house in Paris?"

"What do you mean by small?"

"Somewhere in the range of 50 people would allow us to invite relatives and close friends."

"Works for me."

"After we come back from our honeymoon in the Alps, I have decided not to go back to work in Africa."

"Oh yes, you mentioned this when we were in Geneva last time. I hoped we would be able to be together in Geneva, but didn't think it was fair to ask this of you. Do you want to stop working?"

"No. I plan to talk with my boss about working at the Médecins Sans Frontières (MSF) Headquarters in Geneva."

"What would you do?"

"I looked into what jobs were available there. It looks like I could get a position recruiting nurses to join MSF."

"Are you concerned you might miss the hands-on clinical care you excel at?"

"I probably will, but after being separated from you this year for months at a time, I'm certain I would miss you more. Also, if we decide to have a child this would be a very good position for me to take."

"Do we need to decide now whether to have a child?"

"I think we can hold off this discussion until we get the other pieces of our lives together."

They continue to discuss the wedding and the people they would like to invite. After walking for 45 minutes, they are at the Brooklyn side of the bridge and walk down the stairs to Washington Street and into the historic Dumbo area of Brooklyn. The streets in Dumbo are made of cobblestone. The buildings used to be warehouses, but now are mostly office space, shops and loft apartments with preserved outside architecture from the previous century. They spend time walking through the area and stop for dinner at a wine bar and then grab dessert at the Blue Marble Ice Cream shop. They take the subway back to their hotel and spend the last night together in New York in each other's arms.

The next day they take a taxi to Newark Airport and fly back on the same plane to Geneva. Aceline still has a one-stop flight through Brussels to get to Kinshasa, DRC. "My flight takes off in an hour. I know there is a ton of work you need to do, so you don't have to wait around."

"I am not leaving until you board the plane. I am going to miss you big time."

"Me too. I will be back on December 14 and we can talk on the phone every day until then."

When Aceline gets up to get on the plane, she and David embrace for a few minutes. When they finally let go, there are tears in both their eyes. She hugs him one last time and then boards the plane. David walks out of the airport and gets on bus #28. He goes to his office and tries to get some work done, but is unable to get his mind to focus on anything except Aceline. He gives up after an hour and decides to walk to his apartment to get some exercise and try to clear his head.

Chapter 13

Geneva Switzerland, Winter of 2017–18

David spends the rest of the week going through his emails and snail mail on his desk. One email is from the Director-General, congratulating him on his upcoming marriage and thanking him for the excellent job he did presenting to the UN Secretary-General about the issues arising from the pandemic. The email ends by noting that he has scheduled a meeting with David early next year to hear about the new ten-year emergency plan. This last sentence results in David walking over to Philippe's office. He summarizes what happened at the meeting with the UN Secretary-General. They spend the rest of the afternoon discussing what expanding the five-year plan to a ten-year plan will require. They agree that the five-year plan is still pertinent, but must develop a more comprehensive plan to better prepare for the next influenza pandemic. Philippe offers to work with the influenza experts in their section on expanding the pandemic plan, including how to speed up the development and regulatory approval for microarray patches.

Over the next few months, Philippe and the influenza group work on enhancing the pandemic plan and report their progress on a weekly basis to David. During this time, David is spending most of his time dealing with a new Marburg virus-induced hemorrhagic fever outbreak in Uganda. Marburg hemorrhagic fever is a rare, but serious, zoonotic disease with the first case usually caused by interaction with African fruit bats. The disease spreads between people by droplets of body fluids from those infected or in contact with contaminated objects. Patients present with flu-like symptoms and the mortality rate is around 60%.

As December approaches, his workload still has not lightened, but he knows he promised Aceline he would be at her parents' house the week before the wedding. He talks to Philippe to make sure his absence will not cause them problems. "I'm worried about taking a full week off before the wedding and a second week in the Alps for our honeymoon."

"Our group can handle the work. If I see your face in here after December 14, I will personally call the Director-General's office and get your badge access taken away."

"David laughs. You're a really good friend and I am thankful you agreed to be my best man at the wedding."

"When you are back from the Alps, you will be a married man. As your friend, I will be all over your case if you are spending too much time at work."

***

David and Aceline had discussed having a small wedding of no more than 50 people when they were in New York. However, when Aceline talks with her parents, she finds out that they want to invite additional relatives and friends. After a number of conversations between themselves, they agree to invite 75 people. Aceline and David hope the actual number will be smaller, given that many invitees may have other plans for the holiday season.

David arrives at Aceline's parents' home in Senlis, a small town in the outskirts of Paris. They spend the week hanging out with her parents, Claudette and Alain, and getting ready for the wedding. In France, all couples must have a civil wedding to become legally married. The mayor marries David and Aceline in the Town Hall on December 22, 2017.

The following evening, the ceremony with family and friends takes place in an enclosed heated tent in the backyard of her parents' home. Sixty of the invited people were able to attend along with the minister from the church her parents attend. Snow is falling outside as David and Philippe, wearing sapphire blue tuxedos, walk to the front of the tent. A few minutes later Aceline and her best friend, Bridgette, enter the tent. Aceline is wearing an A-line V-neck sweep train chiffon wedding dress with a split front and Bridgette is wearing a red long one-shoulder dress with ruffles. Aceline had helped David pick out his tuxedo, but he had not seen the wedding gown she is wearing. He briefly wonders why this beautiful, warm, caring and intelligent woman has agreed to marry him. When she gets to the front and turns towards him, his smile runs from one ear to the other.

They told the priest they had written their own vows and at the appropriate time during the ceremony, David would go first. Thirty minutes into the ceremony, the time has come for David to read what he has written.

"I know my lady loves me
For within preoccupied trembling eyes
She allows me to see the beauty deep within her
Sketching fleeting castles without windows
As if there never could be hurt outside
Such wisdom of dreams comforts me
I caress your love when we walk together
Saying few words at times
Anytime something threatens to intrude
You take me inside your heart
To share and dwell with you
I love and believe in you
Forever"

David looks up from his vows and sees shock and love simultaneously expressed on Aceline's face. A moment passes before she can compose herself to read her vows.

"I have never before felt the love we have between us.
I struggle each day we are not together.
Let our feelings for each other continue without diminishing.
I choose you this day to love and confide in, to share with and go everywhere with.
I choose this day to spend the rest of my life with you."

Aceline turns to David who has tears in his eyes. He mouths, "I love you," and they passionately kiss each other. The priest finishes the ceremony and Aceline and David walk past everyone into the house. They go into their bedroom to change clothes for the reception.

Aceline hugs David. "Your vows were beautiful. I didn't know you wrote poetry."

"I started writing when my parents passed away. Somehow, it gave me comfort. I have kept some of them in a book and if you would like, I can share the book with you. I loved your vows and would like a copy of them."

"I can't wait to read your poems."

"While we were getting married, all I could think about is that I am the luckiest man in the world."

"David, I feel the same way."

David embraces Aceline. "If we didn't need to go back to the tent for the reception, I would be ripping off your clothes right now."

"I guess you will just have to wait until after the reception."

Aceline and David walk back into the tent and the band plays the song *Unchained Melody* by the Righteous Brothers. Aceline first heard the song in the early 1990s when she saw the movie *Ghost*. David and Aceline dance with everyone watching. The song ends and Alain takes Aceline's hand for the next dance and Claudette does the same with David.

"David, Alain and I are delighted you are part of our family. We think you make a wonderful couple and everything Aceline tells me suggests you will treat her well. I just don't want her to go through another period of heartbreak like what occurred with her first husband."

"I appreciate your concern. I love Aceline with all my heart and can't imagine doing anything to hurt her."

"That makes me very happy. I know it is presumptuous to discuss this, but we are hoping for a grandchild or two."

"I know Aceline wants a child and we have discussed this several times."

"The way you responded makes me think you are not sure."

"I want to have a child. My concerns relate to our age and our work schedule, but I hope we can make a final decision soon."

"Thank you for sharing your thoughts with me and I promise not to bring up the topic again."

The band continues playing and some of the guests go to the dance floor. David and Aceline mingle among the other people at the wedding. David sees Narendra, who works with him at the WHO, and walks over to greet him.

"Thanks for coming to the wedding."

"I wouldn't miss it. I must admit I never thought you would get married, given how many hours you spend at work."

"Neither did I, but love does strange things."

"Do you know anything about Aceline's bridesmaid?"

"Her name is Bridgette. Why do you ask?"

"She is stunning and appears to be here alone. I'm attracted to tall athletic-looking women, and her long black hair and dark eyes are enchanting. Is she married?"

"Aceline told me Bridgette recently broke up with her boyfriend. Would you like me to introduce you?"

"Yes."

David introduces Narendra to Bridgette and after a few minutes, breaks away from the ongoing conversation. He finds Aceline and they spend the next three hours chatting with everyone. When all the guests have left, they go back to Aceline's bedroom. Clothes fly everywhere and after an hour, they fall into a deep sleep.

***

The next morning, they go out for breakfast with Aceline's parents and then head to the French Alps for their honeymoon. They greatly enjoy skiing, hiking and all the uninterrupted time they are able to spend with each other. On the last day before heading back to Geneva, Aceline updates David on her work situation. "Thanks to you, this year has been the best time of my life. The most important thing for me is for us to be together so I'm going to look for a job in Geneva."

"I came close to bringing up this topic several times this week, but didn't want to pressure you. I know MSF is going to be unhappy, but I am delighted."

"Before I left the DRC, I told my supervisor I was not coming back. She was clearly disappointed, but said she understood. She offered to speak to the Director of Human Resources in the MSF Geneva office and recommend me for a position there. Yesterday, MSF sent me an email, asking me to come interview for a position that is open in their Geneva office. I will set up an interview date for next week and will know more after that."

"Well, I am glad there may be an opportunity for you to keep working for an organization whose mission you care about. Since this is the last night of our honeymoon, I made dinner reservations at <u>Vina Annapurna</u>. Philippe told me he went there last year with his wife and the food was fantastic."

"Sounds wonderful."

Chapter 14

Geneva Switzerland, January 2019

Aceline and David return from their honeymoon at the beginning of January and the following week she interviews for and accepts a job as a recruiter for MSF. She enjoys the work and finds her experience working in Africa gives her credibility with the nurses she is recruiting. David and Aceline both travel for work-related activities about a week per month and try to coordinate their travel so that they are home together whenever possible. While Philippe continues to work with his group on the ten-year pandemic plan, David is overseeing the work of all the other members of the Human Emergencies Program. Even though the workload continues to increase due to several new outbreaks, he leaves work by 5 p.m. whenever Aceline is in town.

David is also arranging a WHO-sponsored meeting with Zika virus experts scheduled for late January. In early December he had sent an email to Venetia asking her to speak at the meeting. Today he heard back from Venetia who indicated she will be at the meeting and Luiz will be traveling with her. She indicates they will arrive several days before the meeting so that they can experience Geneva. He tells Aceline that Venetia accepted his invitation to speak at the meeting and her husband would be traveling with her. Aceline smiles and says, "Wonderful! I'd like to meet them. Why don't we invite them to dinner at our apartment?"

"Great idea."

"Do you know when they are arriving? Oh! And will they bring their baby on the trip?"

"Venetia indicated that her parents happily agreed to care for their son, Julio, while they are away. They are arriving a week from Monday."

"Oh wow. Okay, let's give them a day to recover from their plane trip and invite them for dinner the following evening. What do you think about also inviting Narendra and Bridgette to dinner?"

Her last comment takes David by surprise. "At our wedding, Narendra asked me to introduce him to Bridgette. When we got back from our honeymoon, he told me they had started to date. Have things become more serious?"

"All I can tell you is that Bridgette told me yesterday that she will be coming to Geneva to be with him next week."

"Perhaps I should change careers and go into matchmaking."

Aceline laughs and David winks at her. "You are a funny guy. Having them join us for dinner with Venetia and Luiz should prove interesting and fun."

***

On the day of the dinner, David leaves work early and heads to the market with the grocery list that Aceline gave him in the morning. When he arrives at their apartment, Aceline is already in the kitchen working on the meal. He puts the groceries down and hugs her.

"It looks like you are already hard at work."

"I do love a good dinner party. Before dinner, I thought we would sit in the living room with some champagne, cheese, olives, and almonds."

"Champagne is my specialty. I'll make sure it is ready before they arrive at 7:30 p.m. What's on the menu for tonight?"

"We start with a salmon mousse. The main course is pan-fried chicken cordon blue wrapped in Swiss cheese with a side of broccoli. The dessert will be apple tarts with vanilla ice cream. What wines do we have in the house?"

"A Sauvignon Blanc and a Chardonnay. Do you have a preference?"

"Let's offer both."

Narendra and Bridgette arrive just before Venetia and Luiz. David takes their coats and after the introductions, everyone sits down in the living room. David offers everyone a glass of champagne. "Aceline and I are delighted you could join us for dinner."

"Thanks for inviting us. This is actually the first time we traveled somewhere without our son, Julio, accompanying us."

David asks, "How is Julio doing?"

"As you know, during my pregnancy I was concerned about being infected with the Zika virus, but Julio is almost a year old and developing normally."

David claps his hands. "Well that must be such a relief!"

Luiz smiles. "He looks like Venetia, for which I am grateful."

"Luiz is a proud father who dotes on Julio. I think he has features from both of us."

Aceline asks, "Can we see some pictures?"

Luiz pulls out his phone and passes it to Bridgette. "Venetia, I agree with you. Julio has your black hair and dark complexion and Luiz's eyes and round face."

Bridgette gives the phone to Aceline, who says, "He is beautiful. Someday I hope David and I are blessed with a child."

Aceline had previously discussed this topic with Bridgette but Bridgette hadn't gotten an update in a while. "Have David and you made a final decision about whether to have a child?"

David chimes in, "Aceline and I went to see an obstetrician last week to discuss the risk of a couple our age having a child. She told us that for women over 35 and men over 40 years of age, there is a small increase in the risk of having a child with Down syndrome or another genetic problem. She also discussed the tests that are available to determine if the baby has a genetic problem."

Aceline adds her thoughts. "At this point, we both think the small increase risk is worth the chance to have a child, but are working through whether we would consider having an abortion if there is a problem. Venetia and Luiz, David told me you went through something similar when you were worried Julio might have been infected with the Zika virus."

Venetia takes a minute to answer. "That was a very hard decision. Luiz and I are Catholic and based on our religious beliefs, we decided an abortion was not an option."

Luiz then adds his thoughts. "I favored the decision we made, but would have supported Venetia no matter what she decided. Each day I prayed Julio would be normal, but while he was in the womb, there was no definitive test to answer that question."

"That's a very good point. David and Aceline will not need to wait until their baby is born to know if there is a problem," Bridgette notes.

Aceline sees why David enjoyed his time with Venetia in Brazil so much. The conversation felt open and easy. "I greatly appreciate your willingness to share with us what you went through."

Narendra then says, "Bridgette and I need to discuss if we want children after we get married."

David and Aceline share stunned glances. The room goes quiet for a minute and Aceline breaks the silence. "WOW! I told David I thought Bridgette and you had started to date seriously, but had no clue the relationship had rapidly progressed to the point of discussing marriage."

Aceline's reaction does not surprise Bridgette. "When I came to Geneva this week, Narendra took me for a walk along the lake the first evening. We stopped on the bridge near the Jet d'Eau and there he proposed to me. He later told me he thought I was going to say 'no' because of the look on my face. I actually said 'yes' pretty quickly, but he did not hear me."

"I actually thought Bridgette would say we need to spend more time together before we discuss getting married. All I know is that even when we are not together, I think about her day and night. We have not set a date, but we will likely get married towards the end of this year."

David refills everyone's glass with champagne and gives a hearty toast to Narendra and Bridgette. A few minutes later, Aceline asks everyone to come to the dining room for dinner. The conversation centers on work-life balance.

Aceline has been thinking a lot about how she can successfully mix work and family. "Venetia, how do you find time for yourself and each other with all of your responsibilities at work and home?"

"We hired a woman who stays with Julio on the weekdays until one of us gets home. This woman is amazing and it comforts us to know that Julio is getting good care while we're at work. When at home, we spend our time with Julio when he's awake. We also reserve some time each night for just us. During the weekends, we spend time together doing things we both like."

David follows up, "That sounds like great balance. How did you find the right person to care for Julio?"

"That was a major concern for us. Luiz suggested we used an agency that specializes in finding home care for children. The agency did a lot of the legwork to make sure that the people they sent to us to interview were trustworthy. We wanted someone who had their own children but was now living on their own. We also wanted a person who had done this type of work before so we could talk with their previous employers."

"Makes sense. How do you find time for yourself?"

Luiz answers this question. "We both like to exercise so every other weekday morning one of us goes to the gym and the other stays home until the caregiver arrives. Our parents also come over so we can get out one or two times a week."

Aceline turns to Bridgette and Narendra. "I hope this conversation is not boring you."

Bridgette shakes her head. "I find this conversation fascinating. My mother once told me she was constantly trying to find a balance between her roles as a physician, mother and wife, and at any given time, she felt she was only doing two of these well. Overall, she must have done this well since she and my father are still happily married. I hope I can do the same."

Narendra adds, "This discussion has been helpful and it's clear Bridgette and I need to talk about all of this."

The rest of the evening involves other stimulating discussions and much laughter.

***

The rest of 2018 passes by quickly. Aceline is happy with her recruiting job and David's workload is heavy but he only rarely stays late at work. They spend their evenings experiencing the joy of being together.

After the 2018 Christmas holidays are over, David receives a call at work that the Director-General would like to meet with him in an hour. He asks the Director-General's administrator what the meeting is about, but she does not know. He spends the interim time thinking about what the Director-General wants. He can think of various possible reasons, but none of them seems likely. He walks over to the Director-General's office knowing he will soon find out.

"David, thanks for coming on short notice. This morning, I received a call from Masozi Igwe, who recently took over as Regional Director of the WHO African regional office. She just came back from Ituri and North Kivu in the DRC northeastern provinces where she met with the DRC Health Minister regarding the recently declared Ebola virus outbreak. She was very concerned that this outbreak will be worse than the Ebola outbreak that occurred in the western area of the DRC earlier this year, which was quickly contained. Her concern was due to the lack of trust in the DRC government of those living in the northeastern part of the country. Masozi indicated most of those living in this region were ignoring the Ebola recommendations from the DRC government. She thinks this situation has the potential to be as bad as the 2014 Ebola outbreak in West Africa, where the Ebola virus infected more than 28,000 people and killed over 11,000."

"Yesterday, I heard from one of the people in my group that the DRC government officials were having trouble getting people to come to the healthcare centers and tracing the contacts of those people infected by the Ebola virus. Do you want me to travel to the DRC to determine what else can be done to help get the outbreak under control?"

"I do. We can't let this turn into the fiasco that occurred in Western Africa in 2014."

That night, David tells Aceline about his meeting with the Director-General and that he will be leaving for the DRC in a few days. She is very upset by this news. "David, I think I am pregnant. My periods are very regular and I am now two weeks late. I was going to buy a pregnancy test tomorrow to find out for sure."

David's face lights up. "This is fantastic news. I know when we first talked about having a child, I wasn't sure we should. However, I thought I'd made it clear that I am totally on board." David hugs Aceline tightly but notices she is shaking. Now he starts to worry. "Is something wrong?"

"I knew you would be excited if I'm pregnant. My concern is for you. A substantial number of medical personnel who worked in the 2014 Ebola outbreak became infected and died. In addition, the eastern DRC has many armed groups and innocent people often find themselves in the middle of the conflict. We both have been in these types of situations, but now that we are married and may have a child on the way, I'm really scared."

David embraces her. "I suspect I'd be nervous if you were traveling to the DRC at this point. However, I can't refuse the Director-General's request and I believe the risk to me is very low."

"Why is that?"

"As you know from our time together working in Liberia during the 2014 Ebola outbreak, the virus spreads by direct contact with someone who is infected, and those who are infected are only contagious when they are sick. Unlike previous times when you and I were in the DRC, I will not be caring for patients."

"What about the violence in that part of the country?"

"The Director-General promised to provide me with additional security personnel if I think I need it."

"I realize this is part of your job and I need to be able to deal with it but it is still hard. Will you call me every day?"

"Of course I will. Do you want to take a walk outside and get some dessert?"

"Swiss chocolate and fresh air are just what I need right now."

"Me too. Should we also stop at the drug store and pick up a pregnancy test to find out if we are going to be parents?"

"Great idea."

Later that evening, Aceline comes out of the bathroom holding the test. She is smiling.

Chapter 15

Butembo, DRC, February 2019

David leaves for the DRC two days later taking an 11-hour one-stop flight from Geneva to Kinshasa, DRC. He meets with Dr. Samuel Ngoy, the DRC Health Minister, the next day. David knows Ebola outbreaks are controllable if the government, along with the public health workers are doing their job, and the affected population trusts them. Based on his experience in the 2014 Ebola outbreak in Western Africa , he is also aware of the many things that can go wrong and wants to hear from the DRC Health Minister what he believes the issues are.

Dr. Ngoy thanks David for coming and makes clear he wants to do everything possible to avoid the severe outbreak that occurred in Western Africa. "We know the virus is transmitted when someone has droplet contact with someone who already has symptoms from the disease. The DRC has had multiple Ebola outbreaks during the past five decades and we were able to stop the spread of the outbreak by identifying contacts of Ebola patients and following them for 21 days to determine if they develop symptoms. Why are you having trouble controlling this outbreak?"

"All these previous outbreaks occurred in the western part of the country. The current outbreak is in the eastern part of the country where some of the population does not trust the DRC government. We have sent most of our public health people working in Kinshasa to the eastern region of the country, but many of the people living in the east are refusing to cooperate with those working for the government."

"Can you be more specific about what the population is refusing to do?"

"Of course. Many Ebola-infected patients are refusing to come to the healthcare centers. Instead, one or more family members are caring for them, and some of them become sick. Additionally, when someone dies, the family and others in the village are not following suggested burial practices. This is leading to large numbers of people in a village developing the disease."

"I know the Ebola vaccine was sent to the DRC about six months ago to use in contacts of someone infected with the virus. Is the vaccine helping?"

"Many people are refusing the vaccine. They don't trust anyone they think is associated with the government, including the WHO and non-government groups providing care in the affected areas."

"Do those in the villages where the Ebola disease is occurring understand that the vaccine can prevent them from becoming ill due to the Ebola virus?"

"Our public health workers explain that the vaccine can prevent Ebola, but many still refuse the vaccine."

David wants to make sure that people are being educated about the vaccine. "I actually participated in the Phase 3 study with this vaccine while I was caring for Ebola-infected patients in Guinea during the 2014–16 Ebola outbreak. Over 3,200 doses of this newly developed viral-vector vaccine, genetically engineered so that a harmless vesicular stomatitis virus can express a protein from the Ebola Zaire virus strain, was used in a ring vaccination study where contacts of infected patients were given a single dose of the vaccine immediately (i.e., rapidly vaccinated group) or 21 days after the infected person was identified (i.e., delayed vaccinated control group). The vaccine enabled people to produce an antibody that proved to be more than 90% effective in preventing disease and contributed to ending the outbreak.

"David, our public health staff understand and communicate information indicating that the vaccine has been shown to be safe and efficacious. They are able to convince some people to take the vaccine, but many people still refuse the vaccine because they do not trust what is being said."

Dr. Ngoy and David continue the discussion for several hours. David feels he has a better understanding of some of the issues and decides to head back to his hotel to get some dinner and sleep. He arises early the next morning for his long trip to the area where the Ebola outbreak is ongoing. He flies to the city of Goma in the DRC where WHO security personnel are waiting to take him via a Land Rover on a 9-hour ride to an MSF-run health center in Butembo caring for Ebola patients. He tours the facility with Dr. Pierre Martin who works for MSF and is in charge of this healthcare center. "How many Ebola patients have received care at this facility?"

"Over 100 and most are women and children. This is similar to other treatment centers where almost 80% of those infected in the current Ebola outbreak are women or children."

"Do you understand why in this outbreak the percentage of women and children infected is much higher than in the previous outbreaks in Africa? I recall that during the most recent one in West Africa, the majority of Ebola patients were males?"

"Unlike the 2014 Ebola outbreak, many of those infected in the DRC are not coming to the health centers for care. They are staying in their villages and are cared for by their wives. The caregivers don't have protective equipment and many become infected with the virus. Since many caregivers have children, they can infect their children after developing symptoms themselves. I have seen families where the husband has passed the virus to their wife, who then passes the virus to all their children over a 1–2-month period. It's heart-breaking."

"What percentage of your patients are surviving?"

"Around 35%."

"Wow, I was hoping it would be higher. Have you found any treatment that seems to help?"

"Up until now, there were not any drugs available to decrease mortality. Recently, the US National Institutes of Health developed a specific antibody using the blood of Ebola patients who survived. The preliminary studies with this antibody look hopeful. Luckily, we will be one of the centers participating in a study to see how well it works in infected patients."

"How are the healthcare personnel holding up to the strain of caring for Ebola patients?"

"Approximately 25% of our staff work for MSF and many of them worked in the 2014 Ebola outbreak in Western Africa. The rest of the group is composed of Congolese healthcare workers. A small number of these native staff were involved in previous small Ebola outbreaks in other parts of the DRC. However, this is the first Ebola outbreak in this part of the country and none of them previously experienced an outbreak of this intensity."

"When I cared for patients in the 2014 Ebola outbreak, I found it hard to work for more than an hour at a time because the protective gear covers every inch of your body and it quickly becomes very hot. Has the protective gear become any easier to wear?"

"All of us find it difficult to use this protective equipment and we try not to stay in the equipment for more than 90 minutes at a time. However, we are often short of healthcare workers and end up breaking this rule.

"Has this led to any serious mishaps?"

"Unfortunately, yes. We frequently see healthcare workers develop dehydration on days when the outside temperature is particularly high. Even more concerning, a recently hired nurse violated protocol by taking off her head cover and was exposed to a patient's secretions. We have been monitoring to see whether she develops any symptoms suggestive of Ebola."

"Did she become infected?"

"She developed a fever yesterday after 15 days post-exposure. We put her in an isolation room. Her Ebola test was negative last night, but we are going to repeat it tomorrow as well as do a test for malaria. Hopefully, her illness is not due to Ebola."

"Do you know if healthcare workers in other treatment centers contracted Ebola while caring for patients?"

"When I called the MSF office about our nurse, they noted that Ebola infection of healthcare workers has occurred at other healthcare centers. When I asked how many, she estimated more than 100."

"That is very concerning."

"Yes, and it has made the staff very nervous."

"I noticed some of the tents and storage buildings look like they have been hit with bullets. What happened?"

"Last week, four men armed with guns attacked our center. They burst into one of the rooms and forced people onto the floor before taking their belongings. They then ran out of the building firing bullets randomly. One of the bullets wounded a staff member and damage occurred to several buildings. Things could have been much worse had it not been for one of our staff who was able to send out a distress message — the attackers left when they heard the police sirens. While this is the first militia attack at this health center, other medical sites experienced attacks by other militia groups as well as family members of those who have died from the Ebola virus."

"Do you know who the militia groups are?"

"We think they are members of the Mai-Mai armed forces."

"Who are the Mai-Mai?"

"The term Mai-Mai does not refer to any particular movement, affiliation or political objective, but a broad variety of groups with various motives for fighting. The Mai-Mai is a loose coalition of different domestic and foreign guerrilla groups. Their leaders can be warlords, village leaders or politically motivated resistance fighters. The Mai-Mai are particularly active in the eastern DRC provinces bordering Rwanda and the North and South Kivu area, especially among minority ethnic groups in Butembo. They are a powerful force in the conflict area and the lack of cooperation from these groups poses major challenges for containing Ebola. Furthermore, we are continuously battling misinformation spread by them."

"What happened to the attackers?"

"One was killed, one was captured, and the other two got away."

"Why are the militant groups attacking healthcare centers?"

"The public health people who work with the community tell us the militant groups and much of the population are suspicious of the outside agencies working in the area. When you go to visit various communities later this week you should ask this question to the public health people who will accompany you as well as the people living in the communities."

David finishes touring the medical center and thanks Pierre for taking the time to help him better understand the problems they are facing. The following day, he visits another treatment center staffed by International Medical Corps where he hears a similar story, although they hadn't experienced an attack on their facility. He feels he has a reasonable understanding of the problems the Ebola treatment centers are experiencing. He decides to ask the local WHO office in Butembo to arrange for him to accompany some of the public health people working with various local communities starting tomorrow.

***

Over the next three days, David hears a variety of personal stories from people who chose to care for family member(s) infected with the virus at home, rather than taking them to the healthcare center. They did this for a number of reasons: they were not allowed to stay in the medical center, most infected people ended up dying anyway, and those who died in the medical center were not allowed to be buried in accordance with traditional beliefs. David knew there were medical reasons for following these policies, but the explanations the public health officials gave to those in these villages were not able to convince most families to change their minds.

Further conversations with community leaders revealed a high level of mistrust of the DRC government, which was related to decades of neglect of the communities in the region and the lack of protection from militia groups that pillaged their villages. The leaders also had similar feelings towards the outside groups helping with the current outbreaks because they only "showed up" during severe outbreaks of some of the diseases that impact the village.

On his last night in the DRC, David invites Conny Mabanckou, an anthropologist working in this region, and Dolvin Bokiba, the leader of the public health group in the Butembo province to join him for dinner. They meet at the Issale Lounge in Butembo at 8 p.m. and after ordering from the menu, David explains why the Director-General asked him to come to the DRC this past week, where he has visited, and what he heard. He notes he would like to pose various questions to them and hopes their answers will give him further insight into potential solutions for controlling the Ebola outbreak. They tell him they will do their best to help him.

"What is the background behind the high level of mistrust in the communities against the government?"

Dolvin was born and raised in Butembo and feels he can help answer this question. "The DRC national government is located in Kinshasa in the western part of the country. The government spends most of its money on facilities and programs benefiting those living in or near Kinshasa and often ignores those living in the east."

"One of the village leaders I spoke with said he believed the government introduced the Ebola outbreak into their region on purpose. Why would he say that?"

Conny has visited many of these villages and has a deep understanding of their beliefs. "The DRC has experienced ten Ebola outbreaks during the past 50 years, but none of them have been in the eastern region. Just prior to the DRC presidential election this past December, the government shut down the voting sites in this region, saying that the Ebola outbreak made it dangerous for people to gather at polling sites since this could lead to further dissemination of the virus to others. Many people felt that the government introduced the Ebola virus into the region to use the outbreak as an excuse to stop them from voting while allowing the election to continue in the rest of the country. Other community members perceive the Ebola response as a business benefiting those who are in power."

"Conny, what is behind the distrust of the outside groups that come to the DRC to help treat those who are sick and stop the outbreak?"

"After years of neglect, communities are suspicious of authorities arriving suddenly to deal with Ebola, while malaria, cholera, measles and other infectious diseases have been killing large numbers of people in this area for many years. Most of the population in this region wonders why these outside groups do little to help with these diseases, and then suddenly appear when the Ebola virus outbreak occurs."

"Is this the main reason why so many of those who develop Ebola do not seek care at the medical centers?"

"This is one reason, but an even more important reason is that the outside groups and public health workers from the western part of the country ask the family members to stop providing care for those who are sick and instead take them to health centers where they are isolated from their families. Additionally, the outsiders insist they must change their cultural norms, including traditional funeral burial practices that include touching those who died. The bottom line is they trust their community leaders and healers more than outside groups."

"Dolvin, you grew up here. What is the history behind all the militia groups and the violence they are inflicting on the population in this region and now the outside groups?"

"Militia groups in this region arose over decades due to tensions over land ownership, ethnicity and the political mistreatment from the government. These militia groups frequently attack communities whose people are of a different ethnicity or contain resources they want. The various militia groups not only battle the government troops, but also fight against each other to get control of available resources. The DRC government has troops in this area, but they are often ineffective in stopping these attacks."

"What do the militia hope to gain by attacking the healthcare centers?"

"Probably the most important reason is that they want to show the population that the DRC government is ineffective in protecting them even in the medical centers. The attackers usually don't harm patients or staff, but instead, burn and destroy health center buildings and medical equipment. The UN has now sent in troops to secure the area where the Ebola outbreak is occurring, but the militia see the UN troops as a threat to them, and this may lead to further attacks."

"The various militia groups seem to be having a major impact on the care we can provide and also stop us from preventing new Ebola cases."

Dolvin agrees. "These overlapping conflicts make it difficult to account for and track individuals who come into contact with the disease. Currently, it's estimated that less than half of those infected are identified and, therefore, there is a large number of people sick with Ebola continuing to infect others in the community."

"With so many patients refusing to come to the treatment centers, it seems impossible to stop the outbreak from spreading within the DRC and into other countries."

"People like Conny and I need to find a way to work with the leadership in these communities so that we can overcome this problem, but to date, all efforts have mostly failed. The spread into other countries is also likely with thousands of Congolese regularly traveling between bordering countries. If containment efforts continue to fail, it could spread further across Africa."

David is now visibly upset. "That would be catastrophic. We can't let that happen."

The conversation continues for almost two hours. David has gained further insight into the problems, but is tiring and realizes that he needs to get back to the hotel and get some sleep. "I greatly appreciate you taking time to provide me with the information I need to make recommendations to the Director-General. I am flying back to Geneva tomorrow, but I hope I can call on you again for your insights and advice." Conny and Dolvin agree that they will help in whatever way they can.

David goes back to the hotel and tries to get some sleep before his trip home in the morning. However, his mind is racing as he tries to process all he has learned and determine what they can do to stop this outbreak. He finally dozes off, but later hears gunshots outside his room. He looks out the window and sees armed men heading into the hotel lobby. He hears people screaming and wonders if they are Mai-Mai rebels. He makes a quick decision to stay in his room and lock the door rather than try to escape by the stairway that is at the end of the hallway. He goes into the bathroom and hides behind the bathtub shower curtain. His heart is racing and he hears people shouting on the floor below. He wonders if he has made the right decision and whether there is time to get to the stairwell and head for the rooftop. He thinks about the advice he got from WHO security experts when he first started to work at the WHO and believes they would have told him to escape, and if that was not a viable option, he should try to hide or as a last resort fight the attackers. Just at that moment, he hears a loud noise and he wakes up from his dream. His alarm clock has gone off and it is time for him to shower and leave for the airport. He lies in bed for 15 minutes trying to recover and decides this nightmare is one thing he probably shouldn't mention to Aceline.

On his trip back to Geneva, he begins to formulate the recommendations he will make to the Director-General, but is concerned that they are likely not going to be adequate to control this Ebola outbreak. When he arrives at the Geneva airport, he decides he needs more time to think about the recommendations, and sends an email to his administrative assistant to move his meeting with the Director-General to the following week. After picking up his luggage, he heads home to see Aceline. As he enters the door to their apartment, she runs over and jumps into his arms. "I guess you have forgiven me for going away."

"I'm the one who has to apologize for giving you a hard time."

"Of course not. I know it's stressful. How are you and our baby in waiting?

"Both of us are great and even better now that you are home and we can spend the whole weekend together."

David is now certain that Aceline does not need to hear about the dream he had last night.

Chapter 16

Geneva Switzerland, Spring-Fall of 2019

avid arrives at work the following Monday and finds a note on his desk indicating that his appointment with the Director-General is at 2 p.m. that afternoon. For the rest of the morning, he stays in his office to finish the recommendations for containing the Ebola outbreak. He is extremely concerned about the inability to control the Ebola outbreak in the DRC and how the Director-General will react to what he has to tell him. Around noon, he asks Philippe to join him for lunch in the cafeteria. For the next hour, they discuss his trip to the DRC and the recommendations he is considering making. Based on their conversation, he eliminates several recommendations because they will be very difficult to implement within this calendar year.

He goes to the Director-General's office for their meeting. "David, I know you recently got married and I want to apologize for asking you to go to the DRC on such short notice. I greatly appreciate you going. Have you had time to process what you learned and come up with concrete suggestions for what we can do to help the DRC deal with the Ebola outbreak?"

As David begins to speak his voice cracks. "I hope so. At the highest level, this outbreak demonstrates how difficult it is to deal with infectious disease outbreaks when healthcare systems in the country can't even provide basic healthcare care for their people. Those living in the eastern region of the DRC believe the government favors those living in the west. There is a very high level of community mistrust of the government and outside healthcare organizations. This skepticism has led many people to ignore the advice on how to avoid infection by the virus and refuse the Ebola vaccine. Exacerbating this problem are armed conflicts involving multiple disparate militia groups attacking various ethnic groups in the area. Recently they have initiated attacks against healthcare centers. The armed conflicts make the outbreak even more difficult to control than the 2014 Ebola outbreak in Liberia, Guinea and Sierra Leone in West Africa."

For the next 30 minutes, David provides further details based on his discussions with healthcare workers caring for patients, public health officials attempting to work with people living in Ebola-affected communities, and an anthropologist familiar with the cultures of different ethnic groups in the region. The Director-General feels like he has a sense of the issues. "David, were you able to come up with recommendations to get this outbreak under control?"

"I have a number of recommendations for your consideration. First, we need to appoint one of the people in my group with expertise in Ebola to work full time in the DRC with the government, volunteer groups and community leaders."

"Do you have someone in mind?"

"Salomon Lunda is an up-and-coming star in my group who lived in the DRC for the first 20 years of his life and was involved in the 2014 Ebola outbreak. He has experience with the new Ebola vaccine we used for the first time toward the end of the 2014 outbreak."

"Have you had a chance to discuss this with him?"

"I talked with him early this morning. Most of his family still lives in the DRC and he seems to like the idea. He asked whether there are adequate resources for him to do what is needed and we agreed to meet again this week after I discuss this with you."

"What are your other recommendations?"

"To win back the trust of those living in the region, we need to better demonstrate our concern about the other issues they deal with on a daily basis. Establishing additional health centers closer to the communities and training healthcare workers that speak their language and understand their culture would be a big step forward. While this will take a new infusion of money, it will allow us to better deal with the various other high mortality infections that occur every year, including diagnosing and treating malaria. One community leader told me that in his village, more people died of measles and malaria than Ebola this year. I looked this up and during the first six months of 2019, there were over 2,500 deaths due to measles compared to 1,700 deaths due to Ebola since the outbreak began in the DRC in August 2018. Furthermore, most of the deaths caused by measles occur in children less than five years of age. If we can staff the community health centers with healthcare workers from the local communities and make it easier to get to the clinics, this would go a long way to improving the medical care in the area for preventing and treating infections and other types of problems, including nutritional deficiencies."

The Director-General smiles. "My number one priority is to develop universal healthcare programs that work at the local level. In the end, this will be much more cost-effective than what we are doing now."

"We also need to involve anthropologists who understand the cultures and needs of the different ethnic groups in the Eastern region. By working with community leaders, they can help us overcome the current high level of mistrust in various communities. The tension is most obvious during the burials of Ebola victims. The safe method of burial conflicts with traditional practices and angers those told not to touch the bodies of those they are burying."

"Can the body be disinfected in a way that would then allow the family to touch the body?"

"This could be done, but it would be very dangerous to those involved in preparing the body for the burial. Therefore, we recommend that family members should not wash or clean the body. Only personnel trained in handling infected human remains and wearing recommended protective equipment should touch or move anyone who has died from Ebola. We have found anthropologists are helpful in getting people to accept this message."

"Tell me more about the reluctance of people to receive the Ebola vaccine?"

"This distrust has gotten worse and at times resulted in people in the community, who are not part of the militias, attacking the healthcare workers. The anthropologists can also help us effectively communicate why the vaccine will help save lives and help us recruit people from the region who we can then train to provide healthcare for Ebola patients and vaccinate contacts of those who are sick. This will have a long-term benefit since they can help care for people after the Ebola outbreak has ended and it will provide jobs for people in this area."

"When I previously asked you to come up with a plan to decrease the impact and number of global outbreaks, you suggested using anthropologists. I liked the idea and think this is a good time to see what impact they can have. Do you think they can also help us with the militia groups?"

"This is the most difficult issue to come up with impactful recommendations. If the anthropologist can help us communicate more effectively with the communities, this could result in them giving us better intelligence on where and when the militia groups may strike. Based on prior experience in other conflict areas, unique solutions based on direct dialogue with the various militia groups are required. On occasion, anthropologists have been helpful in negotiating with militia groups and potentially they can find new ways to help us with this problem."

"Given what you know at this point, how likely is it that the Ebola outbreak will spread to other countries?"

"The nine countries bordering the DRC are at risk of the disease spreading to their areas. Some, but not all, of the countries have already implemented screening for Ebola-infected people at the manned border crossings. We recommended that the other countries begin screening. However, many people cross between borders at places that are not guarded, and this means all these countries remain at risk. We need to help all these countries improve their contact tracing, so anyone with Ebola entering a country can be rapidly detected and isolated."

"Is there any other information or recommendations?"

"I think we covered the major points. I will confirm with Salomon his willingness to take the new Ebola position in the DRC and will keep you informed on a regular basis of our progress."

"Please let him know that we will make available whatever resources he needs."

The following week, David meets with Solomon for several hours to lay out the objectives, expectations and support he will receive if he agrees to take on the newly created position in the DRC. Based on the questions Solomon asks, David is unsure if he will accept the assignment. However, at the end of the meeting, Solomon agrees to take the position as long as he can live in Butembo where his family is and that David will be the person to whom he directly reports. They agree that for the first few months, there will be a weekly time set up for them to talk by phone.

David spends the rest of the day with Philippe to catch up on the various ongoing projects in their division. He is particularly interested in the progress made by the group working on the revised pandemic plan and asks Philippe about this. "The influenza group reviewed the current status of global planning and has concluded that the pandemic plans of every high-, middle- and low-income country are inadequate to deal with the next pandemic. Therefore, they are finishing a plan that has specific concrete goals and measurable objectives with timelines for achieving the desired outcomes. This plan is very ambitious and will be difficult to achieve, but they will make clear that not achieving the stated objectives will put the globe at great risk."

"I would really like to read the draft plan."

"I thought you would, so I brought a copy."

"Aceline has some plans for us this weekend, but I will read it next week."

The answer amuses Philippe. "Before you met Aceline you would have spent the entire weekend reading and thinking about the report. I am glad to see you finally developed some balance between work and home-life."

"Me too. I'm a lucky man."

Over the next few weeks, David considers the proposed influenza pandemic plan. He thinks it is exceptional and if fully implemented would be a huge step forward in decreasing the potential impact of a pandemic on global mortality. Furthermore, many of the proposed actions would help decrease the severity of other infectious disease outbreaks. However, based on previous pandemic planning attempts, he knows there are huge hurdles to overcome, including getting the buy-in from all countries and finding the money to finance the plan. He decides he will work directly with Philippe and the rest of the influenza group during the next several months to create a compelling document that he hopes will inspire country buy-in and donor financing.

⁂

Summer is passing quickly and Aceline is due to give birth next week. David meets with the influenza group for the entire day to finish the Influenza Planning document. The plan details the research needed to create innovative tools to provide earlier detection of influenza virus strains that could potentially cause a pandemic, more effective and rapidly produced vaccines, and large quantities of low-cost antiviral medications in sufficient amounts for use to treat those who become ill in all countries. He particularly likes the plan calling for research studies focusing on different ways to deliver the vaccine and drugs to everyone needing them.

David believes countries will vote in favor of the plan, but based on previous experience, he worries how many countries will really take ownership by putting in the financial and human resources needed to execute the recommendations. David considers reviewing the plan one more time but decides to send it on to the Director-General along with a note that he will be out of work on paternity leave, starting next week. He indicates that Philippe will be covering for him while he is out.

Aceline and David spend the weekend in their apartment finishing the conversion of the small room that has his desk into a nursery. By Sunday evening, Aceline starts to have contractions, and the following morning, the contractions are occurring every ten minutes. They head over to the hospital and Aceline gives birth to their son later that evening. They had spent months discussing what they would name him and finally found a name they both liked. They name their son Xander, a name of Greek origin that means "Defender of the People". David holds Xander and a feeling of joy runs through him. Aceline looks at David. "I can't believe we have a child! Today, and of course the day we got married, are the happiest moments of my life."

"I was not sure exactly how I would react, but I am beyond happy."

"I can't wait until we bring him home and the three of us spend time together. I forgot to tell you that last week I got an answer from MSF's Human Resource Department about how much maternity leave I could take. They said I am due at least three months."

"What do they mean by at least three months?"

"The Human Resources Department is currently updating their maternity/paternity policy to increase the time off for new parents. The person I talked with said it may be as much as six months! What did you find out about the WHO paternity leave policy?"

"Interesting. When I spoke to a person in the WHO Human Resource Department this week, she told me the UN recently submitted a newly expanded parenting leave policy to the International Civil Service Commission that oversees Human Resource policies for all the UN agencies, including the WHO. The proposed parenting policy recommendations would be more family-friendly and include increasing the duration of parental leave to 24 weeks to ensure both parents are given adequate time to bond with their child. The UN based this request on recent studies showing better development outcomes for children whose fathers take paternity leave. She also indicated there is child-care support for parents with young children."

"Fantastic. It would be wonderful if we could both be home with Xander for six months. Will the Director-General really let you take six months of parental leave, given all the ongoing outbreaks?"

"I don't know if there are exceptions to this policy. Even if there are, I think he would use the exception only if something as bad as a global flu pandemic occurred. Hopefully, MSF will expand their maternal leave policy to six months too."

David and Aceline take Xander home from the hospital the following day. Xander becomes the center of their attention and each day is a revelation as they watch him grow and develop. They promise each other that they will not lose sight of their relationship. When Xander is asleep, they enjoy their time together and are still able to find time for some of their individual pursuits that include jogging for Aceline and woodcarving for David.

The first few months of parental leave fly by. David had wondered if he would be able to forget about work and is surprised how infrequently he thinks about that part of his life. He wonders if Aceline feels the same. "Do you realize how little we talk about our jobs since Xander was born?"

"I do. Before I went on maternity leave, I told my boss I was not going to look at emails and that she should call me on my cell phone if she needed me. I have cherished this time and love being able to focus on Xander and you."

"The last day at work, I emailed the Director-General telling him I would be out for 24 weeks. I told Philippe I wouldn't be looking at emails, but he will call if we need to talk. I think Philippe considers it a badge of honor not to interfere with my leave. I'm not surprised he hasn't called, but I am shocked by how little I think about what is going on at work."

"Are you okay about that?"

"I am. You and I have grown even closer and fatherhood is a wonderful revelation."

"In what way?"

"Before I met you, my focus in life was totally on work. I can't believe how much that has changed."

"I hope it does not change when we go back to work."

"Amen."

***

Another month passes by quickly and Xander is almost four months old. He smiles and babbles whenever they play with him. Aceline decides it is a good time to ask David about visiting her parents. Claudette and Alain had come to Geneva for a few days on several occasions since Xander was born, but she knows they would like to spend more time with all of them. "Would you be willing to spend several weeks with my parents at their home?"

"Sure, I like your parents and I think it would be great for them to be able to hang out with Xander for a longer period of time. When would you like to go?"

"We could go this weekend and stay for the rest of the month."

David cracks a big smile. "I can tell Claudette and you have been plotting this for a while."

"You think?"

That weekend they drive to her parent's home in Senlis, France. Claudette greets them as they pull into the driveway and lifts Xander out of the car seat. "Look at this full head of brown hair! The smile on his chubby face is beautiful and those blue eyes sparkle. He looks a lot like you did when you were a baby."

"I think Xander has a really nice combination of features from both of us," Aceline responds.

Alain comes out to greet them. "I can't believe how big he has gotten. How much does he weigh?"

"When we took him to the doctor last week, he weighed 7.2 kg. The doctor said he's doing great," David boasts.

"Speaking of doctors, how are you and mom doing?" Aceline asks.

"The pathology results from my prostate surgery showed cancer, but did not indicate the cancer had spread to the lymph nodes. They did my prostate-specific antigen test last week and the level was undetectable. They will be doing the test every six months and as long as the level does not start going up, I should be okay."

"That is terrific. Mom, how are you doing with your arthritis?"

"About a month ago, it got to a point where I was having trouble walking. My rheumatologist decided to add on a new class of drugs, called biologics that affect the part of the immune system causing the disease. This type of drug has been around for more than a decade and substantially decreases the inflammation in many patients, even those with severe arthritis, like mine."

"I heard those drugs can cause serious side effects, including increasing your chance of having a severe infection."

"They can and that's the reason why they tried another drug first. However, I was in a lot of pain and becoming less mobile. My doctor and I agreed that the potential benefit was worth the risk. Since I've been on it, I can get around much better and I have much less pain. They follow me closely looking for early signs of serious side effects but so far, so good."

"I am delighted both of you are doing better."

"Thanks. Your dad and I are doing so well we would like to offer David and you an opportunity."

Aceline looks to David to see if he knows what their offer is. David looks back and shrugs, indicating that he has no clue.

Claudette notices the puzzled look on their faces. "We know David and you have little time for yourselves and wondered if you would like dad and me to take care of Xander for a week while you take off to someplace to spend time, just the two of you. My parents did this for us when you were just a few months old and it was great."

"Are you sure you can do this?"

Alain gives them the thumbs-up sign. "We would love to spend some time alone with our grandson. Our offer is what I like to call a win-win for everyone."

Aceline and David look at each other and accept their offer.

During the next week, everyone is together in Senlis. During this time, Aceline becomes convinced her parents are not only up to the task of caring for Xander, but are looking forward to having some time with him alone. Aceline and David decide to hang out in Paris for a week and then come back to Senlis to pick up Xander and go back to Geneva. The fact that Paris is only 90 minutes away from Senlis helps them feel comfortable spending a week without Xander.

They book a room at the Hotel Du Plat d'Etain in the Marais district of Paris. The area is a quaint and fun place in Paris, with cobblestone streets, stone architecture, hidden courtyards, and great restaurants. Strolling through the area reminds Aceline of pictures of medieval Paris.

Each morning, they start the day by walking to the Place des Vosges. This park, built by Henri IV, is the oldest square in Paris. The park is a true square, measuring 140 m × 140 m and was the first park in Paris opened to the public. The area within and surrounding the park is breathtaking and is the inspiration for many other squares around Europe.

They spend their week visiting various parts of the town, including the Musee Picasso, which is located in an elegant mansion. This museum contains many of Picasso's art works, including paintings, sculptures and photography. They also visit La Maison Europeene De La Photographie, one of the best photography museums in Europe, Jardin des Tuileries, and a variety of other shops. They dine out most nights in open-air cafes and one night cruising down the Seine River. Every evening, they call Aceline's parents to find out how Xander is and then catch up on the romantic side of their relationship.

Towards the end of the week, David is sitting at the desk in their hotel room browsing through the emails on his phone and notices a high-priority email from Philippe. When he opens the email, he learns that Salomon Lunda was wounded during an armed attack by the Mai-Mai at one of the health centers he was visiting. Aceline hears him cursing. "David, what's wrong?"

"Solomon Lunda, the person in my group that I sent to the DRC earlier this year to oversee the WHO's Ebola outbreak control efforts was shot by the Mai-Mai yesterday."

"Oh my! Is he okay?"

"Philippe says he required surgery, but is expected to recover."

"Does he have any family in the DRC?"

"All of his family live there and Philippe said they are visiting him in the hospital."

"Is there anything we can do?"

"Philippe emailed me because he knew that I would want to know, but indicated that he will call Solomon daily and let me know if there is anything we can do."

Aceline knows that David is upset and now is not the time to revisit the question of him traveling to dangerous places but at some point, they will need to have this discussion again.

After another day in Paris, it is time to pick up Xander and head back to Geneva. When they arrive back at Senlis, they have lunch with Aceline's parents, who are sitting on each side of Xander who is strapped into his highchair. Claudine does not seem to be saying much and Aceline wonders if her mother has something else on her mind. After lunch, they pack up and are ready to say good-bye. Claudette is holding Xander. "We have another proposition for David and you to consider."

Aceline looks at her mom. "Given your last proposal, I can't wait to hear this one."

"Anytime you both need to be away from Geneva due to work, your dad and I would be happy to come there and stay with Xander."

"I can tell you had a great time with Xander and we will definitely take you up on this offer. Dad and you can also come visit anytime you want when we are in Geneva."

"We would love to, but there is not enough room in your apartment for all of us."

"Interesting that you say that. David and I talked about getting a bigger apartment or house but decided to put off looking until after Xander was born. This gives us a great reason to begin the search. In the interim, Dad and you can stay at a hotel as you did when you came to Geneva previously. This will allow you to hang out with us except when you are ready to turn in for the night."

"Good point. Your mom and I will look at our calendars and send you some potential dates. You can choose which works best for David and you."

"Perfect and thanks again for taking such good care of Xander this week. He's lucky to have such great grandparents."

***

A few days after returning to Geneva, David and Aceline start looking for a new place to live. Over the next month, they look at various apartments and houses and their decision finally narrows down to a 3-bedroom apartment near where they currently live or a 4-bedroom house with a nice back yard that is further away. They love the house, but it adds an extra 20 minutes to their daily commute for work.

They eventually choose the 3-bedroom apartment and they move there just over a month before their parental leave is over. Aceline comes up with an idea about what they might do during this final month of leave. "This move has been exhausting. Before we have to return to work, what do you think about taking a vacation with Xander? We could rent a house somewhere and invite my parents to come for part of the time."

"I love that idea. Where would you like to go?"

"Maybe somewhere on the eastern side of Lake Geneva that is quiet."

David pauses, "I was hoping to catch up on emails and other work-related activities the week before I go back to work."

Aceline frowns. "Does that mean 'no'?"

"Have I ever told you 'no'? We can do the vacation and still come back a week prior to our start date. Will that work for you?"

Aceline hugs David and he stares into her eyes. "You must think you have me wrapped around your finger."

Aceline says with a wink, "I don't think, I know. To be fair, Xander and you are in my heart at all times."

"When you first came to visit me in Geneva, I promised we would go to Montreux on the eastern side of Lake Geneva, but we never made it there. What do you think about renting a house in Montreux? It's about 100 km from here."

"What's it like in Montreux this time of year?"

"Cold and peaceful. Given all that we have done lately, I think it would allow us to chill out before we start work. We can hike along the lakeside and the Gorges-du Chauderon valley, visit the Old Town area, and sit and stare at the snow-covered mountains."

"Sounds like heaven to me. I think my parents will love this idea."

"We can drive to Montreux. Your parents can drive or take a train there."

***

The first week of vacation in Montreux allows David and Aceline to unwind from their move. The house they rented has a porch facing the mountains and they sit outside every morning with her parents and Xander, drinking tea and relaxing. David and Aceline take advantage of having "built-in babysitters" and go out on two nights to take in a concert and a movie.

When her parents go home after ten days, Aceline and David take daily hikes along the lake and Gorges-du Chauderon with Xander along for the ride in their child-carrying backpack. The vacation has allowed them to slow down and they are delighted they have another week before heading back to Geneva.

However, on December 15, David gets a call on his phone from his administrative assistant, Marion. "David, I am so sorry to disturb you on your paternity leave, but Dr. Richard Huff at the CDC requested I find you and gave me his number for you to call. I told him you were on leave, but he said he really needed to talk with you. He sounded very concerned."

"Did he say what it was about?"

"I asked, but he wouldn't tell me."

David has a worried look on his face. "Thanks for letting me know. I'll call him now."

David knows this can't be good news. He tells Aceline what just happened and says he needs to call Richard before they go out to dinner. He puts on his coat and walks outside onto the porch. He calls Richard who immediately answers the phone. "Richard, my administrative assistant said you needed to talk with me urgently."

"David, I am really sorry to disturb your paternity leave, but several things have happened that suggest there may be a serious new infectious disease outbreak in China. Last week, I received a phone call from one of the people working in our Beijing office. She told me that Chinese colleagues in the city of Wuhan alerted her about a large number of people in that city developing pneumonia requiring hospitalization."

"China has a lot of influenza cases this time of year. How do they know it is not due to that?"

"She doesn't believe this new outbreak is due to influenza. There are a few cases that test positive for influenza, but most of those hospitalized have tested negative for flu."

"Do they have any idea what might be causing the pneumonia?"

"The Chinese government has denied there is any problem, but patients have overwhelmed the hospitals in Wuhan. I have talked with various colleagues in China and they are very concerned that the pneumonia may be due to a new strain of coronavirus."

"What are they basing that concern on?"

"They indicate the illness is similar to what they saw in the early 2000s when a new coronavirus showed up in Asia and caused the Severe Acute Respiratory Syndrome, or as we better know it, SARS.

"Did you speak to the Director of the Chinese CDC?"

"I did and he would neither confirm nor deny there was a new disease in Wuhan. I offered any help he needed, including sending some of our most experienced people from the respiratory disease branch in Atlanta. He said he would get back to me, but to date, I haven't heard back from him."

"What have the CDC staff members in China been able to find out?"

"We have very limited staff in China. Based on what they have learned they are also very concerned."

"I thought you had a substantial number of CDC personnel living in China and working with their Chinese counterparts."

"We did. However, after the 2016 election, there was a dramatic reduction in our budget forcing us to reduce staffing, including many of our epidemiologists and other healthcare experts, in China and other countries. Those left in China are based in Beijing and our capacity to assess what is happening in other areas of China is hindered."

"Are you worried this could be the start of a new pandemic?"

"I am not sure, but the background noise suggesting something major is occurring gets louder every day."

"What do you need me to do?"

"The relationship between China and the United States is pretty strained right now. It would be helpful if you could find out from your sources what's going on. It would be even better if the Director-General could get the Chinese government to let some of your experts into Wuhan."

"I can't believe we may potentially be on the verge of another pandemic, just ten years after the 2009 influenza pandemic. I'll head back to Geneva tomorrow and talk to the Director-General about getting permission to enter the country. Based on previous experience, it may take a while to get permission from the Chinese government to send in outside experts. In the meantime, I'll also try to find out more from other sources we have inside China."

"David, I greatly appreciate your help. If possible, please see if the Chinese government will allow you to include one or more experts from our group."

"I'll get back to you as soon as I know more."

David heads back inside the house and he tells Aceline about his conversation with Richard. She can see he is very upset and after a brief discussion, they agree they will drive back to Geneva tomorrow morning, cutting their vacation short.

Chapter 17

Geneva Switzerland, Winter of 2019–20

Dav12 drops Aceline and Xander off at their apartment and tells her he will bring the luggage up when he gets back from work. He drives to his office and calls the Director-General's assistant to ask if he can meet with him on an urgent matter. She tells David he is out of the country, but will get in touch with the Director-General as soon as possible. A few hours later, the Director-General calls David, who briefly summarizes his discussion with Richard. The Director-General agrees to contact the Chinese leadership to obtain more information about the outbreak and ask for permission to send a WHO team to China.

Very little information is forthcoming from the Chinese government, despite the Director-General's efforts. Over the following week, David and his group are able to contact various Chinese colleagues they know, and their level of concern increases every day. As Richard Huff suspected, the disease is due to a new coronavirus and the outbreak may have started in one of the live outdoor Wuhan markets. Thousands of people in Wuhan and the surrounding Hubei Province are ill, many hospitalized with pneumonia and some are ending up in intensive care units on a ventilator. There have also been deaths, but how many is not yet clear.

David thinks back to 2002 when a new coronavirus strain (SARS-1) appeared in Asia, causing a severe acute respiratory syndrome with a mortality rate of around 10%. Ten years later in the Middle East, another new coronavirus strain caused a similar syndrome — Middle East Severe Pneumonia (MERS) — that had an even higher mortality rate of approximately 30%. Transmission of these coronaviruses is through the respiratory route. Public health workers were able to eliminate the SARS outbreak, but outbreaks of MERS continue to occur, mainly in various countries in the Middle East.

David is very concerned about whether they will be able to limit the spread of this newest coronavirus. He decides they need to start working on a plan to stop this virus from spreading further. He walks into Philippe's office. "I think the likelihood this new coronavirus will cause a worldwide pandemic is very high."

"I'd like to tell you I disagree, but I am also very concerned. It's frightening that the coronavirus that had caused only mild respiratory tract infections in humans, during the last two decades has mutated in ways that have caused much more severe diseases including SARS, MERS, and now this new coronavirus outbreak. The latest coronavirus is spreading rapidly between people and we now know the Chinese government is obviously very concerned."

"Is there new information indicating an increasing level of concern?" David asks.

"I learned earlier today that the Chinese government is trying to stop the spread of the virus to other provinces outside of Hubei by totally shutting down travel between Hubei and other areas in China. In Hubei, they are requiring everyone to stay in their homes and close all businesses, except those that are essential. Exceptions allow people to go outside their homes for essential needs such as groceries and employees of businesses providing essential services. The fact they are doing this during the Chinese New Year when many people travel to visit with family indicates that the government has a very high level of concern."

"Have you heard anything about the mortality rate?"

"I have heard of figures as low as 1% and as high as 10%. No one seems to have a firm handle on the true mortality rate yet."

"I think we need to create a group to start working on a plan to stop, or at least slow down, this virus from spreading around the globe. I would like for both of us to co-chair the group. In addition to those in our Human Emergency division who have dealt with SARS and/or MERS, we should include others who were involved in the 2009 influenza pandemic. If you think there is someone outside our division who could be helpful, please ask them to participate as well."

"I'll put the group together tomorrow. Do you have a name for this group?"

"There have been three different names given to this outbreak — Wuhan, SARS-2 and Coronavirus Infectious Disease-19 (COVID-19). The first name stigmatizes the Chinese and other Asian populations. In some instances, this has resulted in incidents of violence directed at people of Asian descent. The origin of the SARS-2 name is based on the similarities between the 2002 SARS-1 respiratory disease outbreak in Asia and the current one. I prefer using 'COVID-19' to describe this outbreak since it is easier for people to understand that it is different than SARS-1 and does not lead to discrimination against a group of people."

Philippe thinks about it for a minute and then shakes his head. "I didn't think about the stigma issue, but you're right. The 1918 influenza pandemic was labeled the 'Spanish flu' and this resulted in problems for some people of Spanish ethnicity."

Initially, the lack of data coming out of China hinders the work of the COVID-19 planning group. On January 12, a research group in China published the genetic sequence of the COVID-19 virus and this is helping the WHO and other public health and scientific groups to start working on plans to develop tests to detect the virus, drugs for the treatment of those infected, and vaccines to prevent the disease.

***

Many countries are asking the WHO to provide guidance on how to stop the spread of the virus and treat those who become ill. The Director-General knows there has not been enough time for the COVID-19 group to finish their plan, but asks David to issue some preliminary recommendations. Based on what they learned from the SARS and MERS outbreaks, his group comes up with guidance on how to detect the virus and manage those who are ill. They also make recommendations on the use of personal protective equipment, including gowns, gloves and masks for healthcare workers caring for ill patients.

The first case of COVID-19 detected outside of China occurs in Thailand on January 13. By the end of the month, there are 7,818 total confirmed cases worldwide. Most cases are in China, but 82 cases have occurred in 18 other countries across four continents. A senior WHO delegation has obtained permission from the Chinese government to come to China to assess the situation and exchange information. By mid-February, a WHO-sponsored joint mission, consisting of experts from ten different countries, including the United States, has been able to spend time in Beijing, Wuhan and two other cities. Two members of the WHO COVID-19 group are part of this mission. They interact with health officials, scientists and health workers, and the information obtained gives David and his group a much clearer picture of what is going on.

***

David and others in the COVID-19 group have been working overtime to finalize a plan. He thinks they have made a lot of progress and sets up a time to meet with the Director-General the following day. He knows his family time with Aceline and Xander has suffered since returning from their vacation. He feels terrible about this and decides to head home. When he enters the door of their apartment, two big smiles greet him. Xander is sitting on the floor, and David picks him up and tosses him up in the air several times. Xander squeals with joy.

David walks over to Aceline holding Xander in one arm and gives her a hug with his free arm. She looks at his eyes and sees that they are bloodshot. "David, you look exhausted. I thought we might go out for dinner, but I think it would be better if I warm up some leftovers."

He hugs her even tighter. "I am going to nominate you for the wife of the year."

David plays with Xander while Aceline prepares dinner. After they eat, he reads Xander a story and puts him to bed for the first time in over a week. He comes back into the living room and sits down on the couch next to Aceline. "I'm really sorry our family time has taken a major hit for the last few months."

"I know the coronavirus outbreak is making things crazy at the WHO. At MSF we are busy making plans to recruit new nurses and divert some of our current nurses to Italy where the outbreak is now exceeding the ability of their medical system to care for all those requiring hospitalization."

"How is your recruiting going?"

"I'm spending a lot more time with each of the nurses I am trying to recruit. They have a lot of questions about the risk of getting infected and right now the answer to this question is not really known."

"Does Italy have enough protective equipment for all the nurses?"

"No, and this is scaring off some of the nurses I'm trying to recruit. Furthermore, for those nurses that already work for MSF and have now agreed to work in Italy, I have to recruit additional nurses to replace them in their current positions. I am working more hours each day than previously. Fortunately, Luca is fine with staying with Xander until I get home and appreciates the extra money she earns."

"Hiring Luca to care for Xander is one of the best things we have done. How are you holding up?"

"I'm okay, particularly because I think what I'm doing will help save the lives of people infected by this virus."

"It never ceases to amaze me that so many healthcare workers are willing to put themselves at risk by going into an outbreak where we don't have a vaccine to protect them from getting infected or treatments if they get sick. Your recruiting position with MSF is very important and your previous work in Africa gives you extra credence when you recruit."

"We both put ourselves at risk when we took care of Ebola patients in West Africa. When you went to the DRC last year and I was pregnant, I thought a lot about whether I would be willing to put myself at risk again. I didn't have an answer to this question then, but I do now. My answer would be 'no'. Xander and you have changed the risk-benefit equations for me. How about you?"

"I understand exactly what you are saying. When I went to the DRC this last time, I didn't feel I was putting myself at anywhere near the same level of risk as I did in 2014."

"I agree with that, but you still haven't answered my question."

"Xander and you would make me a lot more hesitant to go. Before this, I would have been one of the WHO people that went to China to learn about the COVID-19 outbreak. My risk tolerance has definitely decreased. However, given my job, I can't promise you that I will never have to travel to an area of increased risk."

"Fair enough."

"Are most of the nurses agreeing to go to Italy, where COVID-19 is now causing thousands of cases, married with children?"

"It's a hard question for me to answer since many of our nurses aren't married or their children are now adults. What is clear is that most of the nurses who decide not to go list their family as the number one reason. How are things looking with your COVID-19 plan?"

"We've made substantial progress with the plan. When the Director-General finally got permission from the Chinese government to allow us to send a few people into their country, we were able to get a better feel for how the virus transmits between people and what we might be able to do to slow the spread of the disease across the globe. The rapidity of the spread in China and now in some of the other countries makes it imperative we get our plan up and running very soon if we are to have any chance of avoiding a pandemic."

"When are you presenting your plan to him?"

"He will be back in Geneva tonight and I have an appointment scheduled for tomorrow morning."

"Then I need to let you get some sleep."

***

David leaves the apartment before Aceline and Xander wake up and arrives at the Director-General's office for the meeting. The Director-General is already in his office and invites David inside. "David, I'm sorry we had to meet this early, but the rest of my day is already booked."

"No problem."

"Before telling me about your plan for the coronavirus outbreak, it would be helpful if you catch me up on where things currently stand."

"Based on the information we have obtained, the number of people infected, hospitalized and dying is much greater than the confirmed cases reported by the Chinese government."

The Director-General's brow furls. "What makes you say that?"

Several people working for the Chinese CDC, as well as physicians and nurses working in the hospitals, tell us that many of the patients are cared for in outside temporary tents. We also observed large numbers of caskets outside some of the hospitals."

"What is the government doing to deal with this?"

"They are building temporary hospitals with thousands of beds. They've also effectively shut down the Hubei Province."

"Wow. How have they done that?"

"The government severely restricted travel throughout the Hubei Province, including in the main city of Wuhan, where over 11 million people reside. They have put in place strict orders for everyone to stay at home except to shop for groceries and do other essentials activities. On top of this, they've shut down all non-essential businesses."

"Has the shutdown been effective?"

"It appears to be. Recent evidence suggests these steps have substantially decreased the intensity of the outbreak."

"I spent the last few days meeting with various European leaders who are very nervous since the virus is now causing infections in some of their countries."

"Based on what we are seeing in Italy, their anxiety is well-founded. The outbreak is spreading like wildfire and is inundating their hospitals, particularly the intensive care units, with severely ill patients. The mortality rate in Italy appears to be higher than in Asia."

"Why is that?"

"To answer your question and to help explain the plan we are proposing to slow down the coronavirus outbreak, it would be helpful to provide you with an update on what we know about the epidemiology of the disease and its clinical manifestations."

"Please do."

"There are now over 89,000 confirmed cases and 2,900 deaths reported in 64 countries. Most of these have been in China, but the number of deaths in Italy and Iran is rapidly increasing.

Yesterday there were 1,800 new cases reported and almost 90% of these cases are from countries other than China. Eleven of the cases are from countries that have not previously had patients with this disease.

These countries span four continents, including Asia, Europe, North America and South America."

"How rapidly is the virus spreading?"

"The spread of the virus between people is pretty rapid. The transmission rate appears to be approximately 2.5, indicating that, on average, each infected person is infecting more than two other people. This transmission rate is substantially higher than seasonal influenza, which is around 1.3, and until it falls below 1.0, the outbreak will keep expanding."

"Do we know why the transmission rate is so high?"

"We don't know what genetic mutation in the virus caused the high transmission rate, but one thing that is becoming clear is that the virus can spread from infected people who are symptomatic, infected people who are not yet symptomatic, and those who are infected but never become symptomatic. Initial evidence suggests a substantial number of those who become ill have acquired the virus from asymptomatic people."

"Do we know what percentage of people who are infected contract the virus from those who never become symptomatic?"

"We posed this question to several of the Chinese public health people tracking the virus and they believe it is at least 30%."

The Director-General is startled. "This high rate of asymptomatic people passing the virus to others is very surprising. Is there any other respiratory virus where so many of those infected acquire the virus from asymptomatic people?"

"This is unusual. All viruses seek out new targets so they can create new progeny by replicating in the host's cells. However, this virus is particularly good at this by being stealthy and using asymptomatic people to transmit the virus and thereby spread the disease. The asymptomatic people feel good and therefore are able to socialize more and thereby interact with more people."

"You said that some asymptomatic people eventually become ill. Can you tell me more about this?"

"The asymptomatic people can be divided into two groups. Some asymptomatic people do become symptomatic and we call them the pre-symptomatic group. They appear to be infectious a few days before developing symptoms. The pre-symptomatic spread of the virus occurs with a number of different microbes. In contrast, a substantial proportion of transmission of this disease comes from asymptomatic people who never develop symptoms. It is the high number of cases caused by this latter group that is so unusual."

"When the number of deaths due to the virus is divided by the number of confirmed cases, it suggests a case fatality rate of around 3.4%. Is it really this high?"

"The infectivity fatality rate is likely closer to 1%. This number is determined by dividing the number of deaths due to the virus by the total number of people infected, including all symptomatic and asymptomatic people infected by the virus. The reason why we can't determine the actual infectivity fatality rate at present is that we don't really know how many people the virus has infected. This is because many of the asymptomatic and milder cases are not seeking care and are therefore not counted. However, this lower-case fatality rate is still approximately ten times higher than seen during seasonal influenza. If we can't find a way to slow down the number of people getting infected, hospitals in many countries are going to be overrun with patients and there will be many millions of deaths."

The color drains out of the Director-General's face. "Are there particular groups that are prone to severe disease?"

"Overall, about 80% of those who develop symptoms have mild to moderate disease, and this group is mainly comprised of otherwise healthy adults less than 65 years of age. They usually present with a fever, cough and body aches. Some have pneumonia detected on an X-ray or CAT scan, but most don't develop severe respiratory difficulty. A small percentage of those infected with the virus present with GI symptoms, including diarrhea, and some of these people develop respiratory symptoms a few days later."

"What about those who develop severe disease?"

"Approximately 20% of those who develop symptoms go on to have a more severe form of disease 7 to 14 days after the onset of their symptoms. This group tends to be the elderly and/or younger adults with underlying chronic medical conditions, including obesity, hypertension, diabetes, cardiovascular disease, pulmonary diseases, or who are immunocompromised. Many of these patients have bilateral pneumonia-causing respiratory distress requiring hospitalization for supplemental oxygen and supportive care. Some of these patients end up in intensive care units on ventilators."

"Do all the patients ending up in the intensive care units have chronic conditions?"

"I just reviewed the data from Italy where the hospitalization and mortality rate is the highest of any country to date. The average age of those hospitalized is 63 years and almost all of those dying had one or more of the chronic underlying conditions I mentioned. While most deaths were due to respiratory disease, the main problem was cardiac failure in some patients. We think the heart is another organ the virus can infect."

The Director-General tells David about someone he knows that recently became ill. "One of my friends became infected with this virus a week ago. He developed shortness of breath and told me it felt as though someone was pushing on his chest and not allowing him to take a full breath. Yesterday, his wife called to tell me he is in the hospital intensive care unit on a ventilator. Do you know how many people requiring ventilator support survive?"

"Can you tell me how old he is and if he has any chronic diseases?"

"He's 45 and I am not sure if he has any chronic diseases."

"Most people his age survive, especially if they don't have chronic diseases."

"That's good to hear. His wife also asked me about their two children who still live with them. My understanding is that children are the least impacted age group. Is that correct?"

"Children and teenagers get infected but only a small percentage develop severe disease. To date, there has only been one documented death in a child less than ten years of age. A small number of teenagers have developed the severe disease but almost all of them had underlying chronic conditions."

"Do we know why children don't seem to get this severe disease?"

"There are a number of hypotheses on why this is true, but no one really knows."

"Can you give me a timeline of what happens when someone is first infected with the virus?"

"When the virus enters someone's respiratory tract, the average incubation time before symptoms develop is around five days, although the range of time can be as short as a few days and as long as two weeks. The symptoms worsen over about a week, but then the fever tends to abate and they start feeling better. Most people recover after that, although their cough can last for weeks to months. However, in some people, the fever reoccurs after a day or two, and they redevelop the shortness of breath and feel sick once again. Many physicians feel this is a signal that the person is now developing severe disease."

"David, thanks for the update. I could go on for another hour asking questions, but I have a meeting in 30 minutes and need to hear about the plan you are developing."

"I'm happy to do so, but need to ask you a question before we begin. I noticed you have not yet declared the COVID-19 outbreak a pandemic. Why is that?"

"I realize at this point the outbreak fulfills the WHO criteria for declaring a pandemic. However, based on what has happened in China and South Korea, if governments can get their people to stay in their homes, we might halt the spread of the virus. Do you agree?"

"I think it is very unlikely. The Chinese govern with much greater control over its population than most other countries. They essentially shut down the economy in the Hubei province for several months to stop the spread of the virus. I worry many of the other countries wouldn't be willing or able to do this."

"What about South Korea? They stopped the spread of the virus without forcing people to stay at home or shut down their economy."

"The South Korean government had the advantage of seeing what was going on in China for almost two months. They used this time, along with the advanced technological capabilities of their private technology companies, to produce the large number of testing kits needed to track people who are exposed to those who were infected. Additionally, their public health system is robust and has a large number trained of people who are capable of tracking contacts of those who are infected. Many countries don't have the public health capacity needed to do this."

"Can you tell me more information about what South Korea did?"

"While South Korea had the second-highest number of cases early on in the COVID-19 outbreak, most of the initial cases could be traced back to a single church group whose members recently traveled to China. At the peak, there were over 900 cases in one day, but widespread testing of people with symptoms, intense tracking of their contacts, quarantining those infected, and broad support from their citizens for these measures, allowed the government to greatly reduce the number of new cases. These capabilities allowed South Korea to avoid inundating its hospitals and intensive care units with sick patients. Unlike China, they did this without imposing severe restriction of movement or substantially impacting their economy."

"Why can't we do this in other countries?"

"Very few countries have the capacity to rapidly produce or acquire the enormous number of tests to do large-scale testing, perform contact tracing, and isolate infected patients, which are the actions needed to stop the spread of the virus. For example, the US is having major problems with producing or acquiring the number of tests they need. They are now at the point where the number of infected patients is too large to think that tracking will shut down the spread of the virus."

"What are you proposing in your plan?"

"For the reasons we just discussed, I don't think most countries will be able to totally shut down the spread of the virus. Our plan attempts to mitigate the rate of spread of the virus using two main steps. When the virus enters the community, people would be told to use social distancing when they are near others who are not part of their household, and if things get worse, then the community would be asked to shelter in place until the number of new cases starts to decrease."

"Does the mitigation policy offer countries flexibility in how to implement the plan?"

"The mitigation policy offers some flexibility by allowing countries to apply these steps in localized areas based on the capacity of the area to care for those who become ill. If sheltering in place becomes necessary, there is also some flexibility built into the plan. For example, countries can allow people to leave their home to exercise as long as they follow social distancing standards."

"What about the use of masks?"

"We note masks as another step that can be added, but right now we don't make this mandatory because we are concerned there is an insufficient supply of masks worldwide. At this point, we feel the masks should be reserved for healthcare workers and others at high risk of coming in contact with those infected with the virus."

"Do we know how effective this policy will be for the COVID-19 outbreak?

"Modeling by public health officials and other experts using a range of transmission rate between 2 and 3 indicates that the plan should result in slowing the spread of the virus between people. This in turn lessens the stress on the healthcare system by decreasing the number of people admitted to hospital wards and intensive care units on any given day. Additionally, slowing the spread of the virus will allow more time to develop drugs to treat the disease and vaccines to prevent people from getting the disease."

"In my meeting last week with European leaders, their greatest concern was making sure we keep a balance between saving lives and affecting the economy. How much will the mitigation process negatively impact the economy of countries?"

"Economists agree that the pandemic is going to have a marked negative effect on the economy no matter what we do. If countries don't mitigate the rate of virus transmission, businesses will stay open longer, but more people will die as the healthcare system is overwhelmed with patients. Some experts who studied the impact of the 1918 influenza pandemic on the global economy believe cities that implemented shelter in place earliest not only had fewer deaths, but their economy recovered faster once the pandemic was over. Finding the right balance will involve using mitigation steps for long enough to avoid exceeding the capacity of hospitals to care for patients, but thereafter easing up on the imposed restrictions."

"You've given me a lot to think about. I realize that if I decide to declare the COVID-19 outbreak a pandemic, it will help your mitigation plan move forward in many countries. I'll talk to my executive team about your plan. I'll also continue to hammer home to leaders of high-income countries the need for additional emergency funding. This funding will allow us to help low- and middle-income countries that are least capable of dealing with the spread of this virus."

***

The virus continues to spread into other countries over the next week and the total number of cases and deaths rise faster than before. The Director-General calls David at home one night and asks him to join him and some other members of his executive team for a breakfast meeting at 7:30 a.m. the following morning. When he gets off the phone, he tells Aceline he thinks a decision has been made about whether to declare the COVID-19 outbreak a pandemic and he will need to leave for work early in the morning to meet with the WHO leadership. "David, do you think the Director-General is going to declare a pandemic?"

"Based on his questions to me, I can't tell. He is trying to balance the impact that declaring a pandemic will have on helping us better deal with the spread of the virus versus the negative impact on the economy of countries."

"It seems to me that even in Geneva, where there are only a small number of cases to date, the economy has already been impacted because many people are worried and staying home as much as possible.

"Do you feel this concern?"

"I guess I do. The last few weeks I have only gone outside to go to work or buy food. Normally, I would have come home and taken Xander for a stroll and shop for anything we need. Now I do any errands before coming home. I have been more cautious, and I have to admit I am apprehensive."

"You're not alone. The Swiss government is contemplating shutting down schools and stores that are not essential."

"If they do this, how long do you think it might last?"

"China has been shut down for several months."

"Oh my God! I hate the feeling of being stuck inside, and not being able to take Xander outside for that long would feel stifling."

"I know. China can do this because the government has very tight control over its population, but I'm not sure that a shutdown for this long will work in Switzerland or many of the other countries."

"If the Director-General decides to declare a pandemic tomorrow, are you going to suggest he recommends that countries shut down for months?"

"I'm going to give him several options, one of which is somewhat less draconian."

Aceline notices that David has yawned several times in the last few minutes. "I could ask you a lot more questions, but I can tell you are exhausted. The thing that you need most before you meet with the Director-General is sleep."

"I think many of the people working with me on the COVID-19 plan are wearing down. Yesterday, Philippe told me he was shattered."

"I hadn't heard that word used in years, but I think it is poignant and describes how many people at the WHO and MSF are feeling. Now off to bed with you!"

He kisses her on the forehead and heads off to their bedroom.

***

When David walks into the Director-General's conference room the following morning, all the members of the leadership team are there. "David, please grab some breakfast from the table. While you're eating, I'll share with you what we have already discussed."

"Thanks. I am very interested to hear what you have decided."

"I have scheduled a press conference for tomorrow where I will declare the COVID-19 outbreak a pandemic. After our discussion last week and talking with people inside and outside the WHO, I think this will help garner the needed resources to better respond to this outbreak. Many, but not all, government leaders agree with attempting to mitigate the rapid spread of the virus despite the potential to accelerate the economic damage that is already occurring."

"What were the deciding factors that made you decide to declare the outbreak a pandemic?

"While unfortunate, Italy provided a powerful lesson about what happens if you don't mitigate the rate of virus transmission. Yesterday, I talked with the President of Italy. He described in vivid detail what has occurred during the past month since the first patient with COVID-19 in their country was identified on February 11. They decided not to enforce mitigation steps to slow the spread of the virus, and now their hospitals and intensive care units are unable to care for all the patients seeking care. They have insufficient quantities of personal protective equipment for their healthcare workers as well as too few intensive care beds and ventilators. Currently, they are trying to develop an ethical protocol to decide who gets on a ventilator and who is left to die. This tragic situation has helped convince the leadership of countries that were initially reluctant to close down non-essential businesses that this and other mitigation steps are necessary.

I am also hopeful that by officially declaring this outbreak a pandemic, it will increase the emergency funding we have requested from high-income countries, foundations and other organizations, which to date, has been insufficient. My leadership team has actually suggested that declaring the pandemic might enable us to utilize 'crowdfunding' where anyone can donate money to help us deal with the pandemic. This is something the WHO has never done before."

David is relieved to hear this. "I believe having the WHO officially declare this a pandemic will help in many ways. The idea of crowdsourcing is very innovative. My group will start working with countries on how and when to use mitigation in their country. I am hopeful that we can apply mitigation selectively to specific hot spots within a country, rather than the entire country. This should help decrease the economic impact."

"Please tell your team we are greatly appreciative of all the work they are doing."

"I will. Is there anything else you need before the press conference?"

"I would like to discuss my speech with you and see if there is anything missing. Can we do that now?"

"Sure."

The meeting ends and David accompanies the Director-General back to his office. "David, I have written a draft outline of my speech that includes the following points:

- "Currently, there are more than 132,000 reported cases of COVID-19 in 123 countries and territories, and over 5,000 confirmed deaths.
- Some countries in Asia, including China, the Republic of Korea, Singapore and Japan, have demonstrated that aggressive testing and contact tracing, combined with social distancing measures and community mobilization, can prevent infections and save lives.
- Europe has now become the epicenter of the pandemic and the virus will not stop there. All countries need to prepare and be ready. Countries must be able to find, test, isolate, and treat every case, to slow down the rate of transmission.
- Every healthcare facility should be ready to cope with large numbers of patients and ensure the safety of staff and patients. Healthcare workers should be able to recognize this disease, provide care and know what to do with their patients. I also want to acknowledge the heroic job all the healthcare workers and others who care for those who are sick are doing. We know this crisis is putting a huge burden on you and your families. We know you are stretched to the limit.
- This is a new virus and a new situation. We all must work together and learn from each other. We must find new ways to prevent infections, save lives, and minimize impact. All countries have lessons to share.
- In the midst of this pandemic, we still must provide for the many other health issues people face all the time. Babies are still being born. Essential surgeries are continuing. People still need emergency care. People still need treatment for cancer, diabetes, HIV, malaria, and many other acute and chronic diseases.
- We are all in this together. Until now, we have been relying mainly on governments to support the response. We thank all those countries who have supported WHO's Strategic Preparedness and Response Plan. However, additional funds must now be forthcoming to help us supply countries with personal protective equipment for their healthcare workers, purchase diagnostic tests, and improve surveillance.
- We must invest to create a unified research capability to develop and test drugs and vaccines. We are calling this the Solidarity Research Program that is designed to enroll people in many countries to test the most promising drug and vaccine candidates. This coordinated

response will allow us to more rapidly determine what interventions will work and equitably distribute them to all countries.

• For those interested in helping to fund this effort, the COVID-19 Solidarity Response Fund, go to who.int, and look for the orange 'Donate' button at the top of the page."[1]

The Director-General looks at David. "I am sure the press will have lots of questions, but do you think I left something out that needs to be in my opening statement?"

"I think you covered the major points but I would emphasize two points. The role of community cooperation is vital not only for mitigating the pandemic, but also for making certain we can provide routine healthcare. In Italy, we have already seen people with other types of healthcare problems, including possible heart attacks and strokes, deciding not to seek care because of fear of contracting the virus if they go to a healthcare center. A different example of care avoidance are parents who don't bring their children into clinics to receive vaccinations and other types of routine care. If this continues, we will have major outbreaks of vaccine-preventable diseases, including measles and polio. The irony of this is that children, who are the group least at risk of developing severe COVID-19 disease, will end up dying of measles or being crippled by polio."

"Great point and that goes back to our previous discussion of the need to utilize anthropologists to communicate with various communities, especially those who don't have faith in their governments."

"I agree, and that brings me to my second point. Research needs to be done, not only to develop better tests, drugs and vaccines, but we also need social and political science research to find ways to increase the cooperation between those making recommendations and the people affected by those recommendations."

---

[1] This is taken from the WHO's Director-General's speech given on March 11, 2020, declaring the pandemic. (https://www.who.int/Director-General/speeches/detail/who-Director-General-s-opening-remarks-at-the-media-briefing-on-covid-19---11-march-2020).

The Director-General agrees and adds another point. "It would also help if we could find better ways to convince people to put their individual desires aside to enhance the public good."

David thinks about two recent conversations he had with friends about what the likely outcome of this pandemic will be. "Recently, I had conversations with two people that relate to your question. I have a friend who is a futurist. He works for a technology company and his job is to make predictions about the future based on current trends."

"What does he say about the pandemic?"

"He believes the world will be a very different place once the pandemic is over."

"Better or worse?"

"He thinks better in the long run. He notes there are already great examples of people caring more about others. Two examples he cited were healthcare workers traveling outside where they live to help in areas with large numbers of very sick COVID-19 patients and the marked increase in the number of people volunteering to work in food banks."

"Nice to hear something positive. Did he give you a prediction about the outcome of this pandemic?"

"No. He told me this is my area of expertise, not his."

"Then let me hear your best guess."

"Yesterday, I talked with Dr. Richard Huff, the Director of the CDC, who has a more pessimistic view of the pandemic outcome, at least in the US. The current administration is ignoring many of the CDC's recommendations on how to mitigate the pandemic. The CDC has detected early warning signs in New York City that COVID-19 may overwhelm their healthcare capacity. He talked to the Secretary of Health, who has dismissed his concerns. In fact, he was told to calm down and stop being an alarmist."

"Governments that ignore the advice of their public health experts do so at great peril. I will make that point at the press conference."

"Thank you."

"You still have not told me what you think the outcome of the pandemic will be."

"I guess the best way I can do this is to compare the COVID-19 pandemic to the 1918 influenza pandemic, the deadliest in history. This coronavirus will infect a large percentage of the world's population, but will be less lethal than the 1918 flu virus. Our ability to mitigate the rapid spread of this virus will have a large impact on how bad things get. I hope my futurist friend is right, because in places where too many people don't care about the welfare of their neighbors, the pandemic will be bad. The pandemic will also be made much worse if too many countries only care about what happens in their own country."

"Just hearing the comparison to the 1918 pandemic sends a chill up my spine. History will judge our efforts by examining how much we were able to decrease the impact of the pandemic on the entire world."

"Hopefully, history will judge us kindly."

Epilogue

This epilogue was written in December, 2020, to update the status of the yellow fever, Zika, Ebola and COVID-19 virus outbreaks described in this book. Additional information on these and other global outbreaks is available at https://www.who.int/csr/don/archive/year/2020/en/.

The February 2016 yellow fever outbreak in the DRC ended 12 months later. During that time, there were over 7,300 confirmed or suspected cases, with 393 confirmed deaths. Since that time, the DRC has not had another yellow fever outbreak. However, multiple other African countries, along with Brazil, have had outbreaks caused by this virus.

The Zika virus outbreak that started in Brazil in April 2015 and spread to other countries in South and North America ended in November 2016. During 2016, there were an estimated 280,000 people infected in Brazil and a large increase in the number of babies born with microcephaly. Since then, the number of cases has markedly decreased. The reasons for the decreasing incidence of the disease are uncertain, but heightened awareness of the public regarding mosquito avoidance measures and some level of herd immunity likely contributed to the decline. The decrease in the number of cases has made it hard to study potential interventions against the virus and there are currently no licensed drugs to treat or vaccines to prevent the Zika virus infection.

The 10th Ebola outbreak that began in the DRC in August 2018 was declared over on June 25, 2020. During this outbreak, there were 3,841 confirmed or probable cases, with 2,299 deaths. Over 100 additional cases have occurred since the outbreak was declared over, mainly due to sexual contact between survivors who can have infectious ebolavirus in their semen for six months or longer, and their sexual contacts who have not been vaccinated. On June 1, 2020, just as the 10th Ebola outbreak was ending in the eastern DRC, the 11th Ebola outbreak in the DRC began in the western Equator Province. The 11th Ebola outbreak was declared over on November 18, 2020. During the outbreak, there were 119 confirmed cases and 55 deaths. Health authorities were able to vaccinate more than 40,000 contacts of those infected and this had an important role in controlling the outbreak. The FDA licensed this Ebola vaccine on December 19, 2019.

The Zika and Ebola virus outbreaks helped call attention to the fact that infectious diseases can severely affect the health of pregnant women and their offspring. This was an important factor resulting in the formation of the Pregnancy Research Ethics for Vaccines, Epidemics and New Technologies (PREVENT) committee to provide guidance for including pregnant women in vaccine studies. This group has published 22 recommendations that hopefully will help ensure that pregnant women across the globe have access to safe and effective vaccines in subsequent outbreaks, including the ongoing COVID-19 pandemic (http://vax.pregnancyethics.org/prevent-guidance).

The first wave of the COVID-19 pandemic started in Asia in December 2019. Some of the Asian countries were able to contain the spread of the virus within their country by using a combination of intense testing, contact tracing, and/or lockdown of areas where the virus was spreading. However, by early 2020, the pandemic had spread into Europe, followed soon thereafter by North America, then South America, the Middle East, and finally, Africa. Many of the countries in these other continents did not manage to contain the virus, despite going into lockdown for several months. During this first wave of the pandemic, some of these countries, including Italy and the US, had regions where the number of cases and deaths overwhelmed medical facilities.

The intensity of the first pandemic wave in most countries in the northern hemisphere calmed down before the summer, but by the fall, a second wave was underway. As of mid-December 2020, a few countries are now experiencing a third wave, and there have been more than 67 million confirmed cases and 1.5 million deaths worldwide. The US has the highest percentage of cases (~20%) and deaths (~18%) despite only having 5% of the global population. The data from over 192 other countries can be found at the John Hopkins University COVID-19 Dashboard website: https://www.arcgis.com/apps/opsdashboard/index. html#/bda7594740fd40299423467b48e9ecf6.

While COVID-19 has taken a tremendous toll on the health and economy of countries, there has been some positive news. The mortality rate due to COVID-19 has been decreasing as we have learned how to provide better care for COVID-19 patients. The incidence of influenza A virus disease during 2020 in the southern hemisphere and northern hemisphere has been very low. The reasons for this remain to be determined, but it is likely that social distancing and the use of masks by many people have contributed to the low incidence of influenza. Another positive occurrence has been the development of several COVID-19 vaccines that were developed in less than a year. These appear to be highly effective in preventing COVID-19 disease, particularly severe disease causing hospitalization and death. This is a remarkable achievement since it usually takes decades for new vaccines to be developed and made available to the public. The development of COVID-19 vaccines has occurred due to the hard work and cooperation between the WHO, scientists, vaccine companies, governments, and funding organizations.

Finally, Dr. Robert Sherertz and I will be co-authoring a non-fictional book that will detail the first 18 months of the COVID-19 pandemic. This book will be published by World Scientific Publishing in 2022.

Acknowledgments

I have written several non-fiction books, but this is my first novel. While these two forms of literature are different, I have very much enjoyed writing this novel and hope you, the reader, also liked it.

There are many people who helped me along the way. My wife Cynthia, and children Rebecca, Seth and Melissa, greatly contributed to reviewing different drafts of the novel and putting up with the many questions I posed to them. I owe a large debt of gratitude to Dr. Sara Sinal and Dr. Larry Givner for reviewing the novel and making many helpful suggestions. I also am indebted to my editor Sook Cheng Lim at the World Scientific Publishing Company who contacted me in March 2020 about my willingness to write a second non-fictional book about COVID-19 (the previous book they published for me was *Inside the 2009 Influenza Pandemic*). At that time, I told her I was in the midst of writing this novel and she indicated they were interested in both.

www.ingramcontent.com/pod-product-compliance
Lightning Source LLC
Chambersburg PA
CBHW050640190326
41458CB00008B/2349